NIGHT THOUGHTS
Reflections
of a Sex Therapist

Avodah K. Offit, M.D.

NIGHT
THOUGHTS
Reflections
of a Sex Therapist

JASON ARONSON INC.
Northvale, New Jersey
London

THE MASTER WORK SERIES

Revised edition 1995

Copyright © 1995, 1981 by Avodah K. Offit, M.D.

Library of Congress Cataloging-in-Publication Data

Offit, Avodah K.
    Night thoughts: reflections of a sex therapist / by Avodah K. Offit.
        p.   cm.
    Originally published: New York: Congdon & Weed, 1981.
    Includes bibliographical references and index.
    ISBN 1-56821-458-8
    1. Sex therapy. 2. Sex (Psychology) 3. Hygiene, Sexual.
    I. Title
    RC556.O326 1995
    616.85'830651—dc20   94-45758

Manufactured in the United States of America. Jason Aronson Inc. offers books and cassettes. For information and catalog write to Jason Aronson Inc., 230 Livingston Street, Northvale, New Jersey 07647.

To sidney, ken and mike

Contents

Author's Note

FIFTEEN YEARS HAVE elapsed since *Night Thoughts: Reflections of a Sex Therapist* was first published. The time has passed with the usual relative motion—faster the nearer one is to the end. Not much seems to have changed, a least on the surface, except for my offering different modes of perception in novel, *Virtual Love.*

Scientifically, little new has been discovered about our liquid passions, our psychology, our physiology, although the mechanism of male erection has been elucidated more fully. Magical new chemicals have been developed to help it stand firm in all weather. Patterns of pressure and bloodflow in female orgasm continue to bewilder us as do the riddles of attraction and arousal. Where there is new information, I have included it.

Nothing much has changed, superficially, and yet everything is different. AIDS has altered the fabric of our sexual lives, tearing it apart, stitching it more firmly together. Sex is now a grimmer contemplation, bearing not only the seeds of life but also the threat of extinction. In my practice, couples cling together because they fear the virus in the streets more than personal disharmony. Celibacy is an acceptable mode of behavior, no longer provoking questions about mental health. Sex as both male and female aggression—with bearers of the HIV virus knowingly contacting clean victims—is not uncommon. We are living in a new age, but it is not always the world of sibling love for which we had hoped.

I have not written a new chapter on AIDS and sex, but where appropriate, I've suggested necessary precautions. It's not possible for me to be lighthearted or reassuring about the plague. My thoughts on AIDS are translated into sympathy and prayers of comfort for the sick and support for the scientists committed to finding a cure.

I wrote *Night Thoughts* in a more optimistic and sexually adventurous era. As I now reread my lines, it is reassuring to observe that the feelings and values with which I was concerned have not changed. I never encouraged sex without love or awareness of the reasons for engaging in this most sublime and frequently mysterious human pleasure. With whom does one have sex, and why? I have always been faithful to these questions.

Avodah K. Offit, M.D.
October, 1994

AT THE END OF THE DAY, when the last patient leaves my office, I sit and stare at my desk. Straightening it up is too much effort. I save it for morning. I search for my keys under a pile of papers. I locate my purse. The lights must be turned off, the wastebaskets put outside, the burglar alarm set. I lock the door behind me—firmly. The last thing I want to think about at night is sex therapy. I want to set aside all the people and their problems. I want to shut the door on all the dramas of the past hours, the sexual malaise, the inadequacy, hatred, fear, and unrequited love. I want to ruminate on, say, the murmurations of starlings or the exaltations of larks.

I walk upstairs to my apartment. If my husband is home, we have a drink together. He has wine; I have Perrier. My life is too sedentary for the calories of alcohol. Even though I have been sitting so long, I am usually too fatigued by my day to tell him much about it; besides, I have to be careful not to violate confidentiality. I listen to him. We listen to music.

My Perrier and I find our way to the bath. Under a foot of water in my big old tub, I lie back, close my eyes, and try to put it all out of my mind. But the dialogues replay themselves. First the offended people talk. I mentally defend myself. What have I done to injure their sensibilities? Did I say too much? Too little? How will I treat them next time? Could my first patient really have been appalled by the idea of masturbation? How can I best show the patient who was furious at me that her anger was really directed at her mother? Was the male patient upset because I was withdrawing from him or because his feelings for me were growing too intense to tolerate?

So much for occupational hazards. As I add hot water to the tub, I make a mental tally of the day's pain: who might be suffering enough to need a call of reassurance, who needs surveillance, who is likely to act out. Reminding myself that I am a general psychiatrist as well as a sex therapist, I make what I call "bathtub rounds," reviewing my patients at the end of the day.

If no one requires immediate attention, the edge of concern recedes. I smile and observe my smile in the mirror near the tub. I add up the glad news of the day. My harassed young couple was able to sustain a visit from parents and to have sex afterward. . . . I received a check with three gold stars pasted on it from a satisfied husband. . . . A male patient's prematurity seems under control. . . . An inarticulate husband has composed an extraordinarily moving love letter to his wife with passages adapted from erotic stories. . . . I begin to feel better. It's time for dinner. Perhaps I will share some of the good news, appropriately cloaked in anonymity, with my husband.

After dinner, over coffee, my night thoughts begin. About ten years ago, I somehow became addicted to writing. Perhaps it came from a need to figure out what I was doing, even as I was doing it. For sex therapy is a fairly new field, and its practitioners have little precedent to draw on. In my office, both strategy and tactics are up to me—and that means planning, or at least thinking. As I write, I think about my patients' lives, about the lives of my friends, about my own. Sometimes they mingle.

Writing helps me synthesize my experience in a way I can never manage during the daily roil. At night, questions become more abstract. I try not to let them get out of hand. I know I can't answer the larger ones. I simply ask why we behave as we do. Why, for example, do some people thrash about miserably in the chains of their unreleased passion while others feel grateful to be undisturbed by any sexual emotion? What accounts for the patterns of difference I detect between the desires and expectations of men and those of women? Are the differences chemical or cultural? How can people change their sexual attitudes—and should they be asked to?

The questions obsess me; the answers rarely arrive in parallel with the problems. Perhaps tomorrow I will have an insight—or next week. Meanwhile I reflect on the paradoxes. Sometimes I turn to the medical journals to see if science has discovered something new—a drug, a love potion, a fresh understanding of a mystery of the body. The medical school library at Cornell University Medical Center stays open late, especially during exam period, and once or twice a week I go there to browse. Afterward, my husband may meet me for a beer (and a Perrier) at a student pub.

I've been reading about sex almost as long as I've been thinking about it. When I was twelve years old, my father's library of engineering textbooks and my mother's collection of respectable histories were augmented suddenly by nine books, discarded by a neighbor because they had been slightly burned in a fire. They included novels and scientific works dealing somehow with sex. The book jackets were charred, but the books themselves were intact. My father told me to wrap them in brown paper and organize them into our library. It was years before I realized why he'd given me that job.

Thanks to him, during my early adolescence, I came into contact with Edmund Wilson's *Hecate County*, D. H. Lawrence's *Lady Chatterley's Lover,* a manual of sexual positions by an unknown enthusiast, and *A General Introduction to Psychoanalysis* by Sigmund Freud. Perhaps because I was beginning my adolescence and aware of amazing changes in myself, I was especially attracted to the lectures on "the sexual life of human beings and the development of the libido." We did not have any sex education in school, nor were there any books on it in my public library. Freud's wisdom seemed a treasure, even more valuable than the elegance of Edmund Wilson's sentences or D. H. Lawrence's abundant sensuality. It explained matters.

From this avid early reading of Freud, I retained two concepts: that sexual disorders were often actively related to mental disorders, and that the "sexual impulses have contributed invaluably to the highest cultural, artistic, and social achievements of the human mind." I was indoctrinated, stamped, programmed, and determined by a philosophy that I accepted totally. Sex was not only the province of psychiatry but also the source of all that was good in human achievement.

I still believe this. I love Sigmund Freud for what he gave me when I was twelve, although in view of my feminism, I have been obliged to remove him, like any parent, real or spiritual, from his pedestal. But he said, too, that I would have to do that.

Before going to bed, I sometimes wander out onto the terrace to view the night sky. Most of the time I can't see it; the urban incandescence is so bright that no stars are visible. But the windows across the courtyard are glowing. Behind them, people are watering plants, baking bread, fixing radiators, flipping television channels. Other windows are curtained, and beyond them, people might even be making love. Good for them. I wish them well. It's not easy to be successfully sexual these days, and perhaps it never was. I do what I can to help.

On Morning Sex

I ASSOCIATE MORNING sex with camping. Although I have never gone camping, I own a pair of new summer hiking shoes. I fantasize backpacking as a romantic experience the way some people dream of New York: gourmet restaurants, vintage wines, a box at the opera, a carriage ride through Central Park at midnight, and love between silken sheets at the St. Regis. The best part of camping must be to open your eyes in the morning, see the sunrise, the sky, and the trees—and feel the warmth of a lover there with you in your double sleeping bag.

I've been somewhat amazed to find that morning sex is controversial. But it is. As a therapist I quickly learned that, between men and women, the varying biological and psychological clocks occasion few controversies as inflammatory as those provoked by the possibilities of sex in the day's first moments. Many men like it. Many women don't.

It becomes a point of conflict most often in the treatment of impotence. If a man has a problem rousing or maintaining an erection at other times of the day or night for psychological reasons, and he is physically normal, it's often worth suggesting that the couple have sex in the morning, when he is "automatically" aroused. The woman can mount him casually and renew his pattern of sexual self-confidence by degrees. I am always surprised when a woman—"desperate" for the return of her lover's potency—refuses to take advantage of the morning. Pressures of time and habits of cleanliness frequently quell spontaneous passion, but one would think that these inconveniences could be ignored in view of the more urgent desire.

Where do morning erections come from? Perhaps the most important source is good health. Men with diabetes, multiple sclerosis, blocked artery problems, spinal lesions, and other disorders frequently don't have them, or if they do, their erections may become progressively weaker. The absence of reasonably frequent morning erections may signify more than lack of interest. It may be a symptom of serious illness.

One frequently asked question is whether morning erections are caused by a full bladder, as men have always thought.

Indirectly, yes, a prominent urologist specializing in sexual disorders tells me. The stretched bladder wall produces an internal stimulation for erection that is conveyed to the penis through the sacral nerves. In addition, morning erections seem to relate to awakening from REM sleep.

REM stands for rapid eye movement. People in this stage of sleep move their eyes a great deal. The sleep is deep and they are difficult to wake. Many such periods occur during the night. Men have an average of three to five erections a night. These may occur during REM sleep or while having an erotic dream, but the coincidence is not necessary. If a man wakes or is awakened during REM sleep, he will get an erection.

The level of testosterone, the male hormone, in a man's bloodstream is highest in the morning; that might seem to explain morning erections, but it doesn't. Although the testosterone level builds all night long, rising in an extremely complicated synchrony with REM sleep, no one has proved that morning erections are necessarily related to it.

Women also have REM patterns of altered vaginal blood flow, pulse pressure, and possibly clitoral enlargement. However, we don't know exactly how hormone cycles affect female sex drive.

Our Victorian ancestors had superstitions that avoided conflict over asynchronous body clocks. They believed that sexual relations were debilitating, and that coitus in the morning was particularly hazardous to the day's performance. The mind would be drained of intelligence and the body so weakened that any competitive physical or intellectual effort was doomed. Morning sexuality was to be thoroughly discouraged except on those rare days in a man's life when he had nothing of significance to do for his subsistence or self-improvement.

For certain men, the dawn-stiffened member merely reflects a call to the loo. It is inconsequential to their emotional and physical lives, as inevitable as opening their eyes, and they pay no attention to it unless a partner should happen to be interested.

For other men the morning erection is a call for action. Having intercourse as a prelude to the day's work or play is for them a bracing tonic, a guarantee of alertness, a means of achieving freedom from distraction. With his sexual needs realized, a man may approach physical and mental challenges with equanimity. Sexual satisfaction helps to make all of life's other joys attainable and pleasurable. As a regular pattern, it would seem, morning sex most attracts hardworking men—it comes at the time when their energies and hormone levels are highest. Those with less pressured lives are often available and interested in sex at most times of the day or night.

Men do have a more obvious pressure of physiological arousal driving them. Their erections demand satisfaction. Often they consider the night's turning, kissing, and holding as eight hours of foreplay that entitles them to sex before orange juice. Beyond that, one of the reasons people like to live together is to be able to have sex more as a spontaneous gesture and proof of affection than as an event requiring preparation. This may not often work out over the long range, but as a starting idea, it's delightful. Men like to feel loved before going anywhere or doing anything. Perhaps sex in the morning is more a proof of basic desire and warmth than at any other time. Elegant grooming and the perfectly shaven face belong to yesterday. The morning, rumpled and shabby, requires acceptance.

Women do not universally abhor morning sex. Indeed, some prefer sex on awakening beyond any other experience: It may prolong a state of sensual half-sleep and continue the tide of sexual excitement that has been rising and falling all night. Others like the morning as a moment of choice. The erection is there for them, without foreplay or demand. The man neither insists, pleads, nor seduces. They can make love or not. Many women to whom I have spoken, however, seem not to want to engage in morning sex, even though it may contribute to the preservation of their marriages. I have to work with them before I can begin to help their husbands.

Women suffer from excessive awareness of their ungroomed selves. Not only are women self-conscious, but they also have greater grooming needs. Those in our society who have not yet joined the ranks of women oblivious to natural odors require more time to attend to themselves before and after sex.

Women are often uneasy about making love without wearing makeup, even in the morning! They wonder if their mascara is runny from the night before. They consider whether their legs are bristly, or—if dark-haired—whether the pinpoints of underarm growth have begun to show. Is the polish on their fingernails chipped, and when will they have time to repair it if they make love now? Should they douche after brushing their teeth and before making love? Will all the feeling be gone by the time they have rinsed away last night's accumulation of bacteria? Will they have time to douche again before going to work, or should they wear a napkin and allow themselves to drip? If they do wear a napkin, will other men, stray dogs, and sharks be attracted to their odor?

It's all far more complex for a woman than for a man, who merely showers, shaves, and slaps on a little after-shave to wash away all olfactory reminders. Society does not condition women to sex in the morning. Romance is candlelight, gleaming wood, perfume, perfection, a walk under the moon. Fireflies signal romance in summer. In August, we kiss beneath stars. Morning belongs to children and Cheerios.

How to break through the barriers? Weekend mornings are often a start, especially if work can be put aside. When there are children, Grandma ought to take them the night before. If she can't, a lock on the bedroom door is an absolute necessity. Merely being able to stay in bed, to watch the sun come up, to know that there will be coffee and newspapers later, helps. Usually both people have to relieve themselves of bladder pressure; that's a good time to brush teeth. This may end an erection, temporarily, but because it's early morning, the fullness frequently returns as one dozes off and wakes again. Slow pacing is crucial.

Besides suggesting toilet habits, I also sometimes attempt sensual descriptions of the morning, to help women realize that lovemaking has not always occurred only at night. Occasionally my maternal and pseudo-poetic efforts work, but more often we have to consider why the woman may be invested in maintaining a man's impotence, or why the man may not desire a cure. People adapt to their disorders and tend to construct a life-style around them. Disorders can be as difficult to surrender as any addictive habit. Trying to cure them may be as dangerous as starting a new relationship because of the potential for failure. Better for a woman to relate to the misery she knows—an impotent man who sweetly phones her twice a day and comes home at six every night—than to face the hopelessness of the incurable or the philandering of the "cured."

The preference for morning sex among married men has other sources, too. One is yesterday afternoon's liaison with someone else. If a man has extramarital sex late in the day, he is often not particularly lively until the next morning, when a memory or a fantasy may continue to be stimulating.

Women's converse disinclination for morning sex may have the same root. Yesterday's tryst may have required so much deception and exacting preparation that sex today may feel like just so much more work. Sex therapists have to be aware of the possibilities for this hidden agenda before embarrassing themselves by talking about the wonder of mornings at the campsite.

If women are not trying to hold on to a partner's symptom of impotence, and they have their grooming under control, and they are not having an affair, they may still dislike morning sex because it makes them feel like objects. Even if romance is discarded as a goal, efficiency too often replaces it. Sexual efficiency—the technical term for the speed and accuracy with which a male animal can place his sperm within a female's vagina—is a frequent source of study among biologists, but as far as most women are concerned, their morning unions are no time for human experiments of this sort. Which is not to say that many women don't like "quickies," but the man who must dash to catch the commuter train can leave his partner as desolate as the man who has an important business meeting after lunch-hour lovemaking. Women who stay at home can begin to resent morning sex; women who go to work can resent it, too. Both may feel left behind, somehow.

Morning sex between clandestine lovers or new lovers is, of course, a different matter. People who are working their way over the first Everest of their passion tend not to know what time it is; morning may be merely a sexual continuation of the night before. Married lovers' meetings may also take place at breakfast—the time least likely to cause suspicion at home. Morning sex under these circumstances is not generically the same as sex in the morning between accustomed mates. Indeed, one patient of mine was the mistress—in the preliberation days when women didn't have to work in addition to being kept—of a very rich and generous man who was unable to express his wish for breakfast in bed at his highly regulated home. His wife was one of those independently wealthy women who maintain a Spartan image. He supported his mistress so that he might have a sumptuous breakfast in bed with her—and occasional minimal relations.

It seems to me that the morning itself has become more important to people. They tend to use the early hours, rather than sleep them away. They get up and jog or, perhaps, stay in bed and make love. Certainly morning sex, as a concept—as something to consider—is receiving far more attention these days, maybe even the benefit of the doubt. I have heard that some couples make a point of getting to bed early, awakening every dawn, and making love for an hour or more before starting the rest of the day. A good way to stimulate the heart, I think. Almost as good as waking in the forest to the sunrise song of a migrant wood warbler.

On Female Orgasm

EARLY IN THIS era of sexual research, one doctor made a study indicating that the closer a woman was to her father, the more likely she was to be orgasmic during intercourse. Naturally that set me to thinking again about my relationship to my father, as well as the connections between my patients and their fathers.

It's difficult to define closeness. Among the first images I associate with my father are three objects: a slide rule, a surveyor's level, and a triangular ruler with different measuring units marked on each of the sides. These items rested next to the rolls of blueprints in the third drawer down on the right side of my father's English mahogany desk. At home they were the only evidences of his work: supervising the creation of the Brooklyn-Queens connecting highway, which bears a plaque with his name on it. He once told me that he was in charge of three thousand men, and that the city gave him a car and a chauffeur. I never saw the car because he prided himself on being a scrupulous civil servant and always took the subway to and from work;

I also never heard him give an order—with one exception. I was never, never to touch the slide rule, the ruler, or the level.

Somehow, I could draw a thinner pencil line against the fine wooden edges of that ruler than against the metal edge of any ruler I could buy. The inner section of the slide rule moved on seductively soft tracks and created a very satisfying wooden click at the end of each traverse. The texture of the black lines and numbers pressed into the ivory surface of the rule made my fingertips tingle. And I liked watching the bubble in the clear alcohol of the level, as I made it move slowly from one wooden side to the other, like a ship crossing the ocean, all afternoon.

Usually, I wiped off my fingerprints and put the things exactly in place before my father came home for dinner.

Once, when we talked, my father told me that he'd wanted to be a doctor but hadn't been able to afford medical school. My mother says that when I earned my medical degree, my father fell in love with me, although he had disapproved of my medical career as sternly as he had of my having anything to do with measuring instruments. Perhaps he did fall in love with me. After graduation, he took me out to dinner, alone, and asked me how it felt to be a doctor. The satisfactions of this moment were reduced from what they might have been had I not already experienced the love of my husband and my preadolescent boys, as well as adjusted to living without my father's approval.

I believe my father and I had an unspoken closeness based on a similarity of mind. We had a like respect for the scientific disciplines. Our physiques, too, linked us, for our wrists and ankles had the same slender bone structure.

In my practice I have found it to be true that women who were close (one way or another) to their fathers are often orgasmic, and orgasmic during intercourse. Perhaps inspired by my father's instruments, I am also very interested in the measure and balance of things—the physiological parameters of orgasm, for example. Now there's a subject. In the late '70s, vaginal photoplethysmography was a development in the attempt to measure those changes in vaginal blood circulation that are associated with sexual arousal and orgasm. Over the years, other instruments had been used—an "isothermal relative vaginal blood flow" device, as well as a strain gauge to measure clitoral enlargement—but the photoplethysmograph was the newest wrinkle. It consisted of a tampon-shaped probe inserted in the vagina and hooked up to an external polygraph that formed pen strokes on graph paper to record the findings. The way it worked was that a light within the probe shone on the wall of the vagina. Blood moved inside the vessels, behind the translucent tissue. Special equipment (a photoelectric transducer) detected the amount of light reflected from the vaginal tissue, thus indirectly measuring the changing quantity of blood within it.

The amount of blood pooled in the vagina is called the vaginal blood volume (VBV). The pressure of pulse waves due to the cardiac cycle is called vaginal pulse amplitude (VPA). The tentative findings were that when women got excited, as during a sexual fantasy, both the VBV and the VPA increased. When they had orgasms (as well as when they were aroused during REM sleep), VPA increased but, paradoxically, VBV went down. Researchers hadn't yet figured out why blood volume should decrease though pulse pressure increased during REM arousal and orgasm.

In spite of such auspicious starts, little new has emerged from studies of female sexual physiology in the past fifteen years. Different groups have continued to present conflicting evidence on such seemingly elementary subjects as whether or not the temperature of the vaginal mucosa and the blood flow of genital vessels increases or decreases during sexual arousal!

Among important subjects, scientists feel that research on HIV shedding during menstruation and sexual arousal could literally save lives, but not enough has been done to be useful. Other researchers have attempted to elucidate the meanings of the concentrations of sodium and potassium in vaginal fluids, the rates of filtration of vaginal fluid, neurotransmitters in female genitalia, the role of the cervix in arousal, the neural control of the vagina, and in what blood vessels arousal actually causes changes. None of their findings conclusively help our understanding. Nor do we comprehend the brain mechanism for female orgasm.

Scientists variously blame the lack of definitive new information on taboo, lack of funding, and the absence of an animal model for study. It seems unlikely in the near future that our hang-ups about sex research will disappear sufficiently for us to study the process in vivo or to breed the perfectly orgasmic female animal for future research.

In any event, one of the main purposes of all this testing and measuring has been to separate the physically from the psychologically nonorgasmic woman. Specific correlations, however, have not yet been made.

This seems to be as far as we've come in new measurements since Masters and Johnson observed in 1966 that vasocongestion—the filling with blood—of the "vaginal platform" was a sign of sexual arousal. It would be appropriate for Masters and Johnson to receive the Nobel Prize for this pioneer work; it was monumentally courageous to have studied and delineated these unmapped areas of human physiology. But who shall nominate them?

Until 1966, mythologies and superstitions about sex and orgasm flourished. Our knowledge was primitive, virtually biblical. The famous names in sexology—Freud and Havelock Ellis—did not make "scientific" contributions by objectively measuring groups of comparable people. Pioneers, they did their best to describe what they knew or saw. At the turn of the century, Dr.

Elizabeth Blackwell noted that some women experienced tightening in their loins and genital area, a sensation she called a "spasm." Whether or not this spasm was accompanied by an ejaculation was uncertain at the time. Ejaculations did seem likely, considering how often bedclothes were wet from women's excretions. In Germany before World War II, Magnus Hirshfeld began to make extensive scientific studies, but his work was destroyed in the Nazi holocaust of humanistic ideas.

But after thousands of years, at least a few elementary facts about women's genital response have been established, facts easily available to anyone who searched. Why did it take so long? Were women so downtrodden as to be objects of men's complete lack of interest? Were men—particularly male physicians—so frightened of women that they dared not explore seriously? Women have certainly had far too little to say about themselves. (This lack of information about females extended for a long time to the animal world. Females' orgasmic patterns have only been studied in recent decades. One would have thought that evolutionists and students of pleasure, pain, and stress would have mapped these parameters in wild as well as domestic and laboratory animals quite thoroughly long ago.)

Masters and Johnson made other observations about orgasm in that incredible year. The uterus undergoes progressive contraction during orgasm. Just as a penis fills, so a woman's pelvis fills. Her vagina engorges; her large lips fill their venous plexuses; the uterus may grow to twice its size because of all the blood in it. Climax expels immense amounts of blood from the pelvic plexuses. The literal amount of fluid that moves in and out of the orgasmic pool is enough, in some cases, to deprive women of consciousness, the same way that fainting does. This quantity of blood must be great, indeed, and validates the intensity of some female orgasm. It "frequently requires as long as ten to fifteen minutes," said Masters and Johnson, for the deep purple color, due to the amount of blood in the vagina, to return to normal after orgasm.

Masters and Johnson also made that famous—and often misquoted—measurement of orgasmic contraction:

> The contractions have onset at 0.8-second intervals and recur within a normal range of a minimum of three to five, up to a maximum of ten to fifteen times with each individual orgasmic experience.

They told us, too, how distensible the vagina is; although we already knew it could expand to accommodate an emerging baby, we didn't know much, then, about how the inner vaginal walls expand, the vagina lengthens, and the uterus tips upward to make a pooling place for semen during excitement.

Another measurement of interest to doctors related to the strength of pubococcygeal muscle contractions. A California physician, Dr. Benjamin Graber, believed that this "PC" muscle was primarily responsible for orgasm, and the stronger it was, the better. He carried on the work of Dr. Arnold Kegel, who invented the original exercises for strengthening the PC muscle, intended to prevent loss of urinary control after the trauma of childbirth. Doctors may still measure the strength of PC contractions with a "perineometer." As the vagina squeezes a pressure-sensitive device, the force created can be observed and measured on a gauge. The higher the pressure, the stronger the muscle.

What you do to strengthen the PC muscle is to squeeze as though stopping a urinary stream. In fact, you learn the exercise by stopping actual urination in midstream. Then you practice squeezing very hard, as often as the doctor prescribes, holding each contraction to the count of six. In addition to tightening against the urinary stream, you also press or clap your belly to your backside, as though flattening a pipe inside your abdomen. You can do these exercises anywhere, at any time, but it's best to have a regimen.

Urologists gave an added impetus to the campaign for strengthening the PC muscle by developing a device called the "Vagette." This machine galvanically stimulates the PC muscle to contract and get stronger just the way such a machine might be used in sports medicine to treat a damaged calf muscle. The machine makes the muscle work and get strong. Women who could not control their urination were offered an opportunity to use it before considering surgery. They spontaneously reported that their sex life improved!

Urologists today often use a series of weighted balls placed inside the vagina and held there for a time. These are similar in principle to the weights used in Tantric sex for the development of orgasmic capacity. You hold—with your vaginal muscles— the heaviest weight you can while walking about.

Dr. Graber built on the original concepts of Masters and Johnson by suggesting that the experience of orgasm might be related to women's perception of changes in blood volume as their muscles contract and press the blood out. It all made sense: the muscles around the vagina contracting during orgasm along with the muscles of the levator ani sling, including the pubococcygeus. Both men and women perceive these moments of climax as intensely pleasurable.

Some researchers have been claiming for the past fifteen years that certain women who tend to be more orgasmic than others have a specially sensitive "G-spot" located behind the walls of the vagina and may be able to ejaculate from this spot. I remain extremely dubious. I haven't seen any pictures of the organ represented by the spot. Samples of the "ejaculate" to date appear generally similar to urine. If such a spot existed, urologists would certainly be eager to confirm it, perhaps because disinfecting or removing it would be good business. So far, to my knowledge, normal women do not ejaculate.

Women do lubricate, however, sometimes copiously. No glands produce this lubricant. It somehow travels through the vaginal walls as a "transudate" or "exudate," which means that no one knows precisely how it gets across. A simple pressure relationship has been postulated but this seems unlikely because of the rapidity with which psychological factors can cause it to disappear. Studies of this fluid have been made over the years. An older one investigated its "low molecular weight organic constituents." It suggested that many lipids, especially glycerol and stearic acid, increase significantly in the vaginal fluid after stimulation. More recently, aliphatic fatty acids, similar to animal pheromones, have been found, but appear to serve no attractant function. Another older study indicated that the amount of oxygen present in the vagina increases during orgasm because so much oxygenated blood flows through it. What all this means is not precisely known as far as sperm survival and transport are concerned, but presumably the fat and oxygen help. Whether or not the transudate keeps sperm alive, it certainly does increase our pleasure. Masters and Johnson observed that women who continue to lubricate after they have had a first orgasm are most easily aroused to a second.

I began by reflecting about my own father; unlike him, my anorgasmic patients' fathers tended not to come home reliably and peaceably for dinner at night. They did not help, however unwillingly, with math homework, nor did they teach their drowning daughters how to swim, or how not to fall off a bicycle. The fathers of nonorgasmic women in my practice were mostly alcoholic, or traveling businessmen, or deserters, or they died when the girl was young. They left their daughters alone, one way or another.

Such an abandoned girl may grow up with a disorder of desire. She may not wish to have sex under circumstances that would arouse most women, or may not want sex under any circumstances at all. She may have a disorder of excitement in which arousal may be inhibited or repressed. Finally, she may have one of the orgasmic disorders. Her excitement may be sufficient, but she cannot release her climax. Something may also impair or render her insensitive to the orgasm.

The fathers of anorgasmic women may also be tyrannical family men, restricting hours and boyfriends. Paradoxically, the chances of helping a woman with a cruel father are better than with an absent one. Sometimes the cruelty can be translated into sexual feeling, particularly if beating or spanking have left erotic memory traces. Occasionally, permission to fantasize spanking during sex will bring on orgasm. Later the spanking fantasy may recede as the woman becomes accustomed to enjoying sex.

When a woman cannot remember any warm, exciting feelings toward her father, or toward any of his possessions, sometimes we can summon up a therapeutic memory of a father surrogate. In one case, a woman's first orgasms began to awaken her at night after we talked about the weekend visits she had made as a child to an aunt and uncle. She had been allowed in their bed on Sunday mornings. Her uncle's innocent playfulness under a satin coverlet was a powerful erotic memory.

Pornography often helps restricted women, particularly girls brought up in convents. Authorities have so denied normal physical lovemaking to these women that their excitement is mainly psychic. They need a forbidden stimulus: pictures of women having sex, pictures of men's organs that are frightening (and exciting) to see. Physical stimulation may do little, since they have long ago put mental blocks in the way of being aroused through a desire to love, touch, and hold. Though orthodox religion accepts sexual affection, the injunctions against it until marriage often destroy the feeling. The lovers of such women may stimulate them to exhaustion and fail. But a pornographic skit of sex with the delivery boy or the moving man may instantly stimulate the orgasmic reflex. Perhaps this reaction is something like dreaming. After people take barbiturates that put them into a sleep too deep for dreaming, they may make up for lost dreams by having too many when they stop taking the medication. Perhaps when sex is no longer repressed, excitement emerges vigorously in response to the emotionless scenarios of pornography because the first impulses to sexual love have been so profoundly forbidden. I don't possess or supply pornographic materials. A patient may need only permission to enjoy them.

Approaching the nonorgasmic, nonexcitable woman's problem with mechanical instruction has not often been therapeutically effective in my practice. Vibrators, dildos, and other sexual machinery are frequently useless. I try to revitalize such women by researching their past to find possible sources of the erotic life force; I try to help them make connections to the acute joys of early life. Although I do not neglect suggesting that they try the motorized routes to orgasm, these seem not to work in the majority of severe cases.

When vibrators do stimulate psychologically handicapped women to orgasm, they may become dependent on the machines and be unable to move on to human stimulation; but without the vibrator, they might never have experienced orgasm at all. When women possess erotic vitality, they are usually able to advance beyond the vibrator, which is not inherently addicting. It may, however, represent the limit of certain women's orgasmic potential.

The less handicapped preorgasmic woman has an excitement

disorder because she does not know how to reach sufficient levels of stimulation to trigger orgasm. She is a woman who likes sex, who is happy with her partner and becomes mildly aroused. Often a vibrator or an elucidation of masturbatory technique will help immediately because she needs only permission and education.

Excitement disorders, then, consist of inhibition (the feelings have never been experienced) and repression (the feelings once enjoyed are now extinguished). The roster of human discords leading to sexual repression is endless. Disturbance of any kind can cause it. Of particular interest, however, is a new problem that seems to me to be the female equivalent of male psychogenic impotence. Judging from my practice, it is reaching astonishing proportions.

One does not usually think of women as being impotent. Mythology has it that they can always "perform" sexually: A little K-Y jelly, and the tightest orifice is operative. That is not the case. Symptoms of pain, tightness, and dryness can occur even with lubricating jelly, although recent products improve on the old surgical standby. Women can be every bit as impotent as men, though they consciously desire good relations. Their pleasure can start—and stop—as unpredictably and with as much clanking to a halt of the sexual machinery as is caused by any loss of erection.

Many women enjoy sex most when they are in good form, doing well at their work, satisfied with life. When life is not going well, they become depressed and enjoy sex less. Yet a certain type of female impotence seems to occur when they appear to have everything, when the world should be their oyster. It might be called "the new female impotence." The new male impotence was said to be caused by increased female demand for satisfaction. Women's assertiveness was thought to put men down. Now a woman may no longer be able to have a relationship with the man who once commanded submission. Or she may not continue to be able to relate to a man whose authority and self-esteem do not increase to match hers. The forms this struggle can take are many, but unresolved dominance is the key that opens the door to disaster.

A flight attendant had been "on the line" for seventeen years, during which time she had also cared for her aging parents and four children. When the children matured, she accepted a management position in the airline. She rose quickly and soon was functioning as an executive, making quick decisions, arbitrating disputes. She became a boss.

Her husband did not become impotent, however. She did. In therapy it emerged that she could no longer respond as a submissive wife to her husband's requests for dinner, clean laundry, a spotless home, and a social calendar. Even though she loved her husband, her anger at his not recognizing her changed status emerged as being unable to have sex with him. When he hypothesized that she should never have taken the new job because it had disrupted their sex life, she wanted to leave him for his insensitivity to the real problem.

In another case, the woman moved up and beyond her husband's level in the same organization. She literally became his boss. Still, he did not become impotent. Again, she did, for he began to find ways to reduce her—to criticize her new "masculine" wardrobe, to pay attention to the flutters of other women, to lament the "death" of his "beautiful, sweet bird." She felt her femininity withering with her marriage.

At the premarital level, a woman's concerns over her future may impotize her. One young woman recently out of graduate school "couldn't enjoy sex anymore" because she didn't know what kind of man she wanted. Did her identity rest with finding an achiever or someone who had already achieved, or did it reside in doing it all for herself? This constituted a serious conflict that depleted her sexuality; to her sex meant attachment and commitment.

A fourth woman had a husband who rose to become the chief executive in a large corporation after a relatively short time. She attempted to become a corporate wife, but unwillingly because she had not yet established her own working identity. She didn't know who she was. She felt she was insignificant. She became impotent with her husband, though she loved, admired, and wanted to please him. In addition to the "new impotence," the vagaries of our society's concepts of gender roles, success, and failure have created a "new depression" among women who have not found their niches.

Disorders of orgasm itself are rare. Perhaps the most common is the orgasm to which a woman is anesthetic: It occurs, but she does not feel much pleasure. This problem was traditionally identified as psychogenic. Today the emphasis is on physical disabilities, for example, disk problems or other spinal disorders. Sometimes a nonorgasmic woman may have an insensitive clitoris. The nerves that connect the spinal cord to the genitals may be damaged by protrusions or growths. In one such case, surgery to remove a protruding disk restored orgasm. However, women still do inhibit or repress their experience of orgasm as a consequence of one guilty burden or another. Like men, they may delay its onset for fear of losing control. They may also worry too much about whether or not they will achieve it.

Masters and Johnson described "multiple orgasms" in 1966 with the boldness and clarity that characterized all their early work:

> A woman generally maintains higher levels of stimulative susceptibility during the immediate postorgasmic period

than men do. She is usually capable of return to repeated orgasmic experience without post-orgasmic loss of sexual tension below plateau-phase levels of response.

Which is to say, women do not lose their vasocongestion rapidly and can maintain enough excitement to have repeated orgasms.

Masters and Johnson also observed that the subjective experience of orgasm differed from one orgasm to the next. There is little to be contributed that is new on this topic, except that experts have for the last few years made the distinction between "single," "multiple," and "sequential" orgasms, thus describing the subjective differences in women to which Masters and Johnson allude.

The single orgasm is discrete and alone; like an Aristotelian drama, it has a beginning, middle, and end. Most frequently, the single orgasm is intensely satisfying and one wants no more. It may consist of a series of contractions, rapid at first and then with a longer interval between, or it may be one long, deep, all-engulfing spasm followed by a flutter of smaller ones. It may occur in other ways, too. Most women begin their orgasmic life with this experience. I often wonder if they aren't conditioned to do so by their exposure to single orgasm male sexuality as a model.

Multiple orgasm is now used by some authorities to signify a capacity for repeated single orgasms. After a rest period, or a time when a woman is not aroused, the process may begin again and a second orgasm occurs.

Finally, orgasms of major or minor intensity may follow one directly after the other, with brief delay or loss of excitement between them. These are generally called "sequential" orgasms.

Women are not as eager as one might imagine to learn how to have multiple or sequential orgasms. The women who do inquire about increasing their potential are often wary. "Will my lover be threatened if I can have more than one?" "What happens when he gets tired, or has already come, and I still want to go on?" "Can multiple orgasms ruin a relationship?" Women are often sensitive to the possibilities of losing the lover who fails in an orgasmic competition, just the way they may respond to men who don't like to be beaten at Ping-Pong, cards, or academics. And it's quite true that many men do become threatened by women capable of multiple orgasm.

Premature ejaculators generally stay away from them. They develop acute sexual anxiety that they may blame on other causes, or they may try to dominate intensely so that the woman will be grateful to relate to them no matter what their sexual ability.

Retarded ejaculators often like them at first because their repeated experience of orgasm seems to turn difficulties into assets. Initially, retarded ejaculators and women who have multiple orgasms can seem "made in heaven" for one another. When the retardation is a consequence of underlying hostility to women, however, a fierce jealousy may develop. Such men may start to terminate intercourse after the woman's first orgasm with the excuse of not exhausting her, or they may develop an extraordinary desire for passive fellatio. It seems to them so dreadfully unfair that the woman can have so many orgasms so easily, while it is difficult for them to have even one.

Whether or not men without specific functional problems are threatened relates to their interpretation and perception of the sex act. Some enjoy giving as much as a woman wants; others can only be aware of their own desires; still others fatigue themselves in a futile effort to please.

A cautious woman might assess her partner's potential response to multiple orgasms before learning how to have them, but I am not convinced that kind of precaution is worth taking. My bias is to increase joy first and deal with the consequences later. Nevertheless, women persist in their questions. Are there actual physical causes—size of a man's penis, for instance, or style of thrust—for multiple or sequential orgasms, or does that seem to be an emotionally governed experience? What sort of reasons, physical or psychological, are there for women desiring one orgasm as opposed to many, or vice versa? Is there an emotional component that may influence a woman's preference for one of a certain type of orgasm, but more of another? Once women do learn to have, or allow themselves to have, multiple or sequential orgasms, do they seem to become dissatisfied with single orgasm lovemaking? Do women seem to have more orgasms in more loving relationships than in one-night stands?

In sex, any and every response is possible. The feelings between two people, their mental states, their physical equipment—even the state of the national economy—may contribute. Perhaps a few general observations can be made.

A man with a large, heavily veined penis who is capable of sustaining high levels of his own excitement may readily assist a certain type of woman to multiple and sequential orgasms. If, in addition, he detumesces slowly, her repeated orgasmic experiences may be encouraged to continue by the turgidity of his penis and the lubrication of his ejaculate.

Conversely, lithe men with smaller organs may "flutter" women to multiple and sequential orgasms with more superficial stimulation. They may also be able to perform athletic maneuvers such as insertion at various unusual angles to stretch the vaginal lips and promote orgasm.

Most men are somewhere between these extremes; for a woman to respond with orgasmic frequency depends on her innate abilities or her capacity for combining fantasy with specific physical stimulation. In general, the longer a man can sustain sexual pleasuring before orgasm, the more he may contribute to the frequent female response.

Nevertheless, the ability to have multiple orgasms is basically under a woman's control. She simply begins lovemaking again after resting, and another orgasm ultimately emerges.

"Sequential" orgasms may occur in response to male manipulation or to psychic stimulation. Most commonly, a woman may bring them on by performing the PC exercises described earlier to develop orgasmic competence. She may begin at any time from a few seconds to five or ten minutes after an orgasm, since it takes some time to lose the vasocongestion of high excitement. These muscle contractions will encourage another orgasm to come on, and another, and another. Women may also develop their own styles of breathing, writhing, or thrusting to bring on more orgasms.

Wanting more than one orgasm is like wanting more of any other pleasure. If the trip is pleasant, one tries to extend it. If the food is good, one continues to eat. Eventually one becomes tired or satiated.

Emotionally, most women crave reciprocity between deep feelings and multiple orgasms. They desire summing or intensification of feelings; the old metaphor of fireworks going off may refer to the orgasm, or orgasms, experienced with emotion. Sequential orgasms may feel like nothing more than a series of knee jerks, or they can be—to quote an enthusiastic adolescent patient who has them—"like being swept into space by an intergalactic shake-up and hanging on to the one person in the world whom you love."

Some people are uncomfortable with being "carried away" and prefer neat little orgasms; others get sentimental or sloppy; still others manage the elegant experience. Again, it's a matter of character. Women who can't release themselves in love may do so in one-night stands; women who might be horrified by one-night stands develop their abilities in deeply committed relationships. One orgasm with a special man may mean more than twenty with someone who has lost his appeal.

The capacity for multiple and sequential orgasms usually develops over years of practice, although some women possess it intuitively. Yet rarely is a conscious effort made to improve orgasmic capability.

After a time with the same lover, a new experience may occur, or new lovers can lead a woman to a variety of sensations. The unique aspect of this growth is that at any specific point she often cannot envision that a more intense pleasure is possible. Her existing orgasmic ability frequently feels perfect and complete, requiring no improvement. Suddenly a change, a new feeling occurs. She wonders why it could not have been foreseen.

Perhaps emotional growth meshes with various physical experiences to nourish the fullest capacity for high pleasure. Over time, one has sexual relations while appreciating such a broad variety of feelings, both one's own and those of one's lover, that new orgasmic paths and patterns may be inspired. One may have private responses or be stimulated by a sudden reach into another person's eagerness. Or a man may offer himself so totally that orgasms well up again and again in gratitude for his gift. To describe the kaleidoscope of feelings that foster orgasmic diversity is a task best left to the poets.

Extramarital Patterns

I STARTED OUT with a rule. If one partner was having an affair, I couldn't treat a married couple for sexual disorder. This rule was based on early Freudian hydraulic theory: If the libido was coursing through the pipes of love to irrigate another love object, the marital sex would wither and die no matter what I might try to do about it. As I quickly came to discover, however, unless I changed the rule, my practice would wither and die.

Eventually I came to the conclusion that in about 60 percent of the couples I treat, one person is making love to someone else. At least half of those who have sex outside marriage are women. I can usually elicit information about the liaison in the first few sessions by seeing the patients separately; women are slower to tell. Others will not reveal their infidelities until several months after treatment begins, when therapy has come to seem too costly with too little result. In desperation, they confess. Among the "monogamous" 40 percent, I rather suspect, there is a significant number of extremely secretive, if not paranoid, adulterers, who tend to drop out of treatment rather than open up.

As I gained experience, I developed an approach. When I knew about an infidelity, especially the kind that absorbs a great deal of one partner's sexual energy, I often turned my attention to the dynamics of the marriage rather than focusing on the sexual problem. What else could I do? The "faithless" partners, pressed by the demands of unhappy mates, might have been in my office against their will. They were often unable to tell their spouses, who had bravely selected the perils of sex therapy, their feeling that sex inside the marriage would never be as good as sex outside it. I certainly couldn't announce their hopeless prediction to the innocent husbands or wives. Nor could I summarily refuse to treat the couples lest they believe that they were crazy, or that I was. All I could do was work with them, for which there was not much precedent in psychotherapy, nor any book of instruction.

With the deceiver, I had to make a pact. We would meet separately, without the aggrieved. I was to be informed frankly and completely about how it all started, what went on, and what the troubles were. That way I could make some sense of the problems in the marriage and the mood swings peculiar to people who engage in extramarital love.

Soon another dilemma arose. On principle, my loyalty was to the marriage. Occasionally, however, somewhat to my surprise, I found myself regarding the affair as good and necessary, and the partner-at-home as distinctly defective in charm, vitality, or insight, not to mention sexuality. At other times, I felt the beauty of the monogamous person's spirit and the soul-sickness of the wanderer. I wanted to protect the good from the evil, even though psychiatry had long since deleted those words from my vocabulary.

Therefore, the first decision I had to make was that I could not have any automatic investment in keeping the marriage together. This argued with my personal values. Nevertheless, the couple in front of me didn't need my personal values to confuse them. I was only there as a catalyst, to help them find their own way.

The second decision involved abuse. I would not condone emotional or financial sadism if it arose or was there at the outset. If a man was publicly humiliating his wife with his mistresses or his chronological absurdities, or a woman was exhausting a man's resources to support a lover or buy designer clothes in which to meet him, separate individual therapy was necessary. They could not use my office as a stage on which to exhibit their deviance.

With those ground rules established, we could start a therapy that had no preconceived destination. If we landed on a new planet, or found a hospitable star, that would be splendid. Otherwise, we were simply looking for a way to travel well together.

What I discovered en route was that the main question no longer seemed to be whether or not people would have extramarital sex, but rather when the probability of doing so was high. The course of married life, I once estimated, provides at least fourteen predictable times for sexual infidelity to occur. All have to do with loss or stress, either transient or permanent, and represent attempts to cope or adapt. These include any point when a man or woman is

1. deciding on or beginning a career;
2. heavily involved in expansion or success;
3. changing jobs;
4. traveling extensively alone;
5. depressed by failure;
6. bored by monotony or fatigued by dull overwork; and
7. retiring.

When any of these events is occurring in the life of one partner, the other is equally vulnerable to a new relationship, however brief or extensive. Apart from those who believe in monogamy with religious zeal, this leaves only well-balanced, happily functioning, permanently employed, bright-eyed citizens to enjoy security in modern marriage. When one considers that both partners have to be immensely pleased with themselves and their life and work—at the same time—in order not to suffer temptation, and that both must be devoid of any desire to spoil their own success, the chances of monogamy grow very slim indeed.

But more must be considered than one's work life. Family crises and events that are often related to extramarital adventures include:

1. pregnancy and childbirth;
2. the period during which small children receive a great deal of attention at home;
3. times of bereavement, such as the death of a parent;
4. periods of other emotional crisis—a child's accident or a mate's illness;
5. the "empty nest" syndrome, when children leave for school or college;
6. any time in a person's life when she or he confronts the process of physical aging, an awareness that occurs at least in every decade of life; and
7. any time of stress such as moving, buying a home, or any major change in style of life.

Certain of these occurrences fall within predictable time ranges. Perhaps the frequency of the "seven-year itch," which has been statistically documented, is related more to the multitude of stresses that often occur around this time than it is to "boredom." The seven-year marriage frequently presents a picture of a new baby, young children, a move, a husband's concentration on career advancement, a wife's dissatisfaction, and in-law problems. Failure to cope can lead to the panacea of an affair.

The twenty-five-year marriage is another collapsible entity, as two people realize that all the earlier reasons for staying together, except perhaps companionship, have expired.

Beyond circumstance, of course, individual tendencies toward attachment or detachment and personality factors that encourage or discourage bonding affect extramarital sex. Most of us are trained by societal customs to develop looser bonds now than ever before. We may not be raised early on by our mothers but rather by helpers or day-care centers. We are sent as toddlers to school, and often to a variety of schools even before sixth grade. The vast perpetual entertainment of television, books, and movies prompts us to fantasize ourselves in romantic and sexual situations that would have amazed our ancestors. In our moves from town to town, town to city, city to country, we are almost nomadic. Social mobility and ease of transportation remove us, all too quickly, from our traditions. Our parents separate, divorce, meld again, creating new personality factions within the family. Emotionally, we become wanderers. In finding a new sexual partner, we strive to protect ourselves from dying of love lost, or being afraid to try anew. We find ourselves more love, in the form of a new lover. (It is an interesting linguistic sidelight that we do not find new "sexers" or new "eroticizers." Male or female, and if only for a night, an unpaid sexual partner is usually called "lover.")

The question is whether people really have to give up their lovers in order to function better and enjoy sex more in marriage. My profound answer is that I don't know. It varies. Some do, some don't. One thing that often amazes me is how eager many people are to do so, provided they can hope for a reasonably pleasant domestic alliance.

In an ideal progression, even when there is a lover near the picture, I try to bring a couple closer, perhaps by helping them to realize how they have been deserting one another through attention to children, jobs, sick parents, or other responsibilities. They may be shown how anger is a form of insecurity, how flattery is often disguised rage. People who take others for granted may reconsider their values; people who feel that their partners are lost may discover they have the power to retrieve them.

If there is hope for the relationship, working on the dynamics will uncover it. It will also often uncover the source of the sexual dysfunction: the wife who teases, plays games of withdrawal, makes ego-shattering remarks so that her husband is always premature; the husband who sees all reasonable requests as demands and withholds his orgasm from his wife merely because she wants it. An impotizing virago may emerge, or a "sleeping beauty" who expects her husband to have a firm erection while she virtually lies in state. Characteristic behavior in life resembles that in sex.

Extramarital sex may be viewed as a retaliation, a crutch to help a marriage stand, or even a basis for it. It may be a total substitute for married love, an antidote for it, or a simple pleasure like going to the movies. Its particular meaning may come up in therapy, when confession, or discovery, leads to catharsis, revaluation, and restructuring the union to serve its partners' intimate needs. In therapy, I try to help a couple reach that point where they may see working together on their sexuality as an interesting new challenge.

And what about those controversial unseen souls, the lovers? My general view is that they don't necessarily need to be discarded. They may fade away. They may go away. The paradox in my practice is that those marriages most inevitably disintegrate where there is trouble, but loyalty and morality prevent taking a lover to alleviate serious stress. The frustration of living with a cold, asexual, or inadequate person who cannot change, and from whom there is no respite, brings on divorce most effectively.

I am as proud of a peaceful and fair divorce as I am of any tender reunion. In the world where people visit me for sex therapy, which may not be entirely like the rest of the world, the aim is to cultivate the couple's best, most honest feelings, and so reduce their suffering.

Menstruation and Sex

IT SEEMS TO take about six months in treatment for my female patients to menstruate in sync with me. Not that simultaneous menstruation is one of our therapeutic goals; it's just one of those curious bonds that often form between women experiencing rhythms of intimacy. We look haggard, feel bloated, and break out in spots together, like girls exchanging invisible body chemistry when they live together in dorms, where the first studies of menstrual synchronization among women were done.

I've been astonished that this unity with my patients has occurred so often, because we are not body-mates. We are not daily exposed to one another's odors. We do not bathe in the same facilities. We do, however, exchange powerful emotional signals. Maybe that has something to do with it. In any case, the simultaneity makes therapy proceed in interesting sine waves. I am never quite sure to whom any given emotion, any up or down of feeling, belongs first.

As a sex therapist, I try to sort out the physical from the psychological. My questions are: How is sex drive related to the menstrual cycle? What are women's reactions to their cycle? What are men's and women's reactions to menstruation itself?

Being dirty, dangerous, and irrational are the historic qualities associated with menstruating women. As late as the 1950s, scientists were attempting to prove that women gave off "menotoxins" that were believed to cause death to flowers and to rats in which they were injected. As early as Leviticus 15:19, if a man touched a woman during her menses, he was unclean. She had to be "put apart" for seven days. Certain Mexican-Americans believe that if a woman urinates outdoors during her menses, her uterus will be invaded by lizards who will build a nest there; later the victim will give birth to a litter of reptiles.

Bruno Bettelheim and other analysts have claimed that men can envy women's wombs and menses; others have reminded us of early womb worship in fertility cults. But most discussions of women's primary sexual organs seem haunted by the biblical view of the menses as a punishment and the womb a source of evil as well as birth. Early medicine reflected these uncharitable concepts of the womb, with a tendency to blame all a woman's ills and vagaries on her "cycle." One Greco-Roman idea was that the uterus moved throughout the body, causing most of a woman's ailments, especially hysteria. A second-century Greek physician wrote:

> In the middle of the flanks of women lies the womb, a female viscus, closely resembling an animal; for it is moved of itself hither and thither in the flanks, also upwards in a direct line to below the cartilage of the thorax, and also obliquely to the right or to the left, either to the liver or spleen; and it likewise is subject to prolapsus downwards, and, in a word, it is altogether erratic.

When a woman's sexual relations were too infrequent, her womb was thought to dry up and go searching through the body for moisture, fastening itself on the heart, the liver, or the brain, among other organs, and prompting afflictions such as shortness of breath, vomiting, anxiety, pallor, headache, and lethargy. When we blame women's troubles on their "cycle," we are not far from these old concepts.

Today, medicine describes the wandering ovum, the fluctuating hormones, and the tides of blood more clearly and precisely.

The menstrual cycle may be twenty-five to thirty-six days long. Directly after menstruation, the "follicular" phase occurs. A cohort of follicles, or egg sacs, in one ovary begins to mature. One follicle gains ascendancy; the others shrink away. This dominant follicle produces a burst of female hormone, estradiol, which then stimulates the pituitary gland at the base of the brain to produce a surge of LH, or luteinizing hormone. The LH helps to release the ovum from the ovary and "luteinizes" the cells that remain behind. They then become the "corpus luteum" and produce the progesterone that both raises basal body temperature and prepares the lining of the womb to nourish the ovum if it becomes fertilized. If there is no fertilization, the corpus luteum dies and the spiral arterioles, small blood vessels of the uterine lining, contract. This may help to expel the menses.

The main hormones governing this activity are, therefore, estradiol, FSH (follicle stimulating hormone), LH, and progesterone. Two others, 17-hydroxyprogesterone and prolactin, also play an important role.

The initial "surge" of hormones to a high blood level usually takes place in the time immediately surrounding ovulation. This has been thought to occur on the twelfth to fourteenth day after the menses start. A 1980 study of the normal menstrual cycle, however, indicated that two thirds of women's cycles had their estradiol and LH peaks from the twelfth to eighteenth day. One third of normal cycles showed a peak before the twelfth day and after the eighteenth!

Therefore, one third of women may peak in the period that starts as early as the eighth day after menstruation begins. Since peak hormones mean peak fertility, the possibility for pregnancy is high until soon before menstruation starts again.

Somewhat later in the cycle, during the early luteal phase, estradiol falls precipitously. Progesterone usually reaches its peak during the luteal phase and falls sharply prior to the menses.

Hormones, therefore, may climb or fall rapidly at almost any time during the menstrual month rather than within the limited times we are accustomed to assigning them. It follows that if hormonal decline is associated with emotional depression, women can become depressed at almost any time of the month. However, if we do not know what a woman's hormone levels are, we can't begin to try to relate her moods or her sexual excitement to her periods. We have not yet made complete enough studies to correlate fertility, mood, and sex drive, although we suspect there may be a relationship between them.

This vast hormonal variation has nevertheless encouraged speculation on women's behavior. Are women naturally less effective than men because of the monthly menses?

According to one set of statistics, some 52 percent of postpubescent women suffer menstrual pain, and about 10 percent of these are incapacitated for one to three days. If premenstrual discomfort was included, the figure would be much higher.

Strategically, these figures are disappointing and alarming. They are disappointing because one cannot make the statement that the majority of women don't suffer. They do. Though a remarkable woman physician named Clelia Mosher demonstrated back in the nineteenth century that "functional periodicity" was not a disabling handicap that should prohibit females from assuming responsibilities in commerce or the professions, there does seem to be a great deal of "dysfunctional periodicity."

In 1980 researchers with a political bent began to examine women's efficiency during their periods. In Great Britain, one study measured women's effectiveness in rapidly distinguishing colors and shapes and telling odd from even numbers. Women performed most of these tasks with equal ability, menstruating or not. The researchers concluded that menstruation does not interfere significantly with task performance. Still, the high-pain statistics are alarming. They suggest that women's reproductive organs have been medically neglected.

The medical questions concern the nature of illness and cure. To what extent are the vicissitudes of menstruation normal? Which menstrual pains are symptoms that can be alleviated through medical skills? Where is menstrual research headed?

It is a hopeful fact that the problem of distinguishing average, normal, and ideal menses is now becoming a preoccupation of medical statisticians. Pain on menstruation may be an illness like the common cold. Yet we have been assessing women who suffer the "illness" to determine what is "normal"—rather like drawing conclusions about normal hearts from heart attack victims. Recently doctors have begun to determine what "normal" menses are by excluding women from study because they have pain. They also exclude women whose psychological profiles confuse the issue. There are many normal women who ovulate yet enjoy life. Their hormones fluctuate but do not cause depression. They may provide a standard against which to evaluate distress. One of the first such studies to involve a significant number of women—sixty-eight—was presented in Stockholm in 1980.

For women who do have pain, researchers have recently developed new substances to prevent distress. These inhibit the contractions of the uterus caused by prostaglandins, chemicals found in male semen and in female tissue. Now a woman can try antiprostaglandins such as ibuprofen, mefenamic acid, indomethacin, or naproxen to stop or reduce her cramps, where before she had only analgesics and low salt chicken soup. They seem to work for some women, although my impression is that a universal pain-reducing agent has not yet been discovered.

Medicine also continues to search for ways to create ideal menses—painfree, bloodless, yet not interfering with the possibility for pregnancy if desired. As we know, the Pill suppresses ovulation and reduces cyclic pain. Pills or implants that allow menstruation every three months are beginning to interest researchers. On the mechanical side, menstrual extraction—sucking the blood out through the cervix with a vacuum pump—is rarely employed. We could all dispose of our menses in an hour a month. The present state of instrumentation, however, makes the procedure too hazardous for everyday home use, and it has largely been confined to abortion.

Medical treatment for what is now designated as the "premenstrual syndrome" is limited. Doctors now prescribe diuretics, low sodium–high protein diets, analgesics, tranquilizers, and exercise. Some women find these regimens helpful. They do keep one busy enough for a few days to take the mind off those symptoms of body swelling, breast tenderness, and pelvic engorgement that cause us to feel both uncomfortable and unattractive. At least the medical establishment has accepted our discomfort as real.

Perhaps the most mysterious medical question of all is: At what part of the menstrual cycle do women have the strongest sexual desire? Is lust programmed cyclically into our bodies, or is the stimulus mostly mental? Studies are equivocal. Some women indicate that midcycle is their "best time." Probably an equal number of women opt for the premenstrual or the post-menstrual period. Some hardy ladies even seem to prefer the height of menstruation.

A decade ago, *The New England Journal of Medicine* published an article that strongly suggested women had a true estrous cycle—that they were more active during the time when they were most fertile. Previous studies had been based on simple coital frequency. This report paid attention to who initiated! During midcycle women who do not take the Pill appear to initiate sex more often than women who take it. Perhaps women are mammals programmed to want sex most when fertile, after all.

We are only beginning to trace the paths of our "instincts." As we grow older in evolution, we seem to learn more about our primitive selves—how we are governed by factors beyond our control. One of the newer "instincts" that we are looking at involves male response to female hormonal fluctuation. The testosterone present in females may have two peak times: the highest at ovulation, the second highest five to seven days post-ovulation. In a study of eleven women that demonstrated this rise, the greatest sexual frequency occurred at ovulation. An additional finding was that male testosterone—in men monogamously living with their wives—rose along with female testosterone, thus giving the lie to the myth that men are always chemically and biologically at the same level. Male sex drive may respond to female sex drive—a new concept for sociobiologists to ponder.

If men's hormones respond to women's, can a woman expect a monogamous partner to follow her through her cycle and match her desires? If a man too frequently pleads headache or overwork on that individually best day of the cycle, should one suspect that someone else is tampering with the gentleman's hormones and short-circuiting the personal response?

Questions raise more questions that we can't answer. Since other studies have shown the male hormone level to rise automatically after sexual intercourse at any time, we still cannot be certain of much.

Physically, most women make a distinction between the way they feel on menstruation after an ovulatory as opposed to a nonovulatory cycle, if they know about the distinction. Women usually begin their menstrual life with light, easy menses. This gentle introduction may last up to three or four years or more. Perhaps it was intended to give the young human female a chance to experiment with sexual partners without the consequence of pregnancy. Suddenly, nature informs many of us that she means business by giving us *mittelschmerz*, premenstrual tension, heavier flows, and more cramping when we are truly fertile. Some women feel this discomfort from early on; others begin to experience it without warning and attribute it to neurosis or psychic pain. One woman first felt it after divorce. She wondered if she had begun to suffer as a response to the emotional trauma, but I suspect her body responded to freedom with fertility, however painful. Another began to experience painful menses after her first premarital intercourse. Though she wondered if her guilt had provoked the pain, perhaps her body became womanly in response to the possibility for procreation. A large part of my work lies in helping women to define their moods and their sexuality in relation to their cycles, and in so doing, I find out a great deal about who they are.

The emotional states that encourage sexuality appear to be different from one woman to the next and from one time in a woman's menstrual cycle to another. Although the journals have suggested more psychosis as well as more murder and suicide among women near or during their menses, in my practice the most common premenstrual psychiatric symptom is a night of tearful self-pity or abandonment bathos. In the midst of housework, eating, reading, or taking a shower, a woman may suddenly begin to cry at the tragedy of it all, even though there has been no particular tragedy. Rather than rising from some true place within, the emotion settles down on her like a mantle. The woman who suffers premenstrual sadness may then respond sexually to the sort of oversolicitousness that might be embarrassing at another time.

Another common premenstrual feeling is severe irritability. During the waiting time before release, women become tense, critical, and easily enraged. Women who respond aggressively to the discomfort of their full womb may find themselves initiating sex in a rage of lust.

Tension may have other positive effects on sexuality: The narcissistic woman may search out added stimulation as reassurance against feelings of unattractiveness at this time; the dependent may require more intense closeness through sex as reassurance against loss. Women who need punishment for sexual pleasure may feel particularly rewarded by premenstrual distress. Histrionic women may take this time to make more drama out of life than it reasonably contains, and to stage violent partings and tearful sexual reconciliations. My experience with patients is that a woman's sexual response to premenstrual tension reflects the way she deals with discomfort, trust, attachment, and sexual pleasure. Personality—the structure of responses and defenses that we acquire—is the sum of these reactions.

Of course, premenstrual tension may have a negative effect on sex as well, as it does perhaps more often than it encourages union. Mildly paranoid women may spend their premenstrual time worrying about their husbands' sexual wanderlust. They may suffer a siege of anxiety about their own sexual abilities. If a woman tends to respond aggressively to discomfort, she may so beleaguer her husband or her partner that sex, if not the entire relationship, may be ruined for the rest of the month. Women without regular partners may respond similarly to their premenstrual symptoms, although they may more often isolate themselves socially. A woman without a mate can stay home alone if she is not comfortable. She can prevent a new relationship from drowning in the monthly currents of unjustified rage or despair.

A woman's reaction to the menses themselves may be more related to her partner's sensitivities than to the actual flow. Men's responses vary from deep inhalation and appreciation of the menstrual scent to disgust at being once more at the "fishmarket." They may be afraid of being permanently stained, or may revel in the bath of their lovers' rosy flow. Some men insist on towels and wipettes before, during, and after; others fingerpaint their bodies like happy savages in celebration of fertility, life, and love. There are men who approach a menstruating orifice like happy vampires in search of bloody sustenance; others seem to fear being poisoned. The world is full of stoics, too, who state, "It's no obstacle." Reaction is character, a lesson always interesting in its variations. A woman's first lover, her long experience with one singular man, or her traumatic experiences may affect the rest of her sexual life. One woman suffered lifelong humiliation because her first lover had said, "It smells like someone's died in there."

How women feel also depends on whether they choose to see themselves as becoming weak by losing blood, being purified of toxic waste, or excreting the beautiful lining of their precious womb. It's all a matter of attitude.

Some women bleed during their menses as though crucified and under no obligation to be brave. Life is black; they take Fiorinal; they go loudly to bed. Parties, food, and music are all unappetizing. Work is impossible. Their time has come. They commandeer their family's pity, careless of the hidden antagonism that lurks behind the service they receive.

Other creatures fade into an agony of headache and *fin de siècle* vapors for which darkness and cologne serve as comfort. They have "migraines." They stay so long alone in the dark that people begin eventually to whisper and knock at the bedroom door to determine if expiration has occurred.

An Italian patient tells of her unfavorite grandmother's former menstrual habits: "She put the rag on and we all knew to keep away." "Putting the rag on" did not refer to a menstrual diaper but rather to a wet linen cloth tied about the head that served the purpose of announcement. Anyone challenging this battle flag was met with immediate verbal execution, confinement to cleaning the oven, or a stint at beating the carpet.

To determine whether this behavior is psychiatrically abnormal or not, one needs merely to look at the rest of the time. Between bleedings, are they free, high-spirited, vital women who stride through their days in charge of life and love? Or are they self-pitying, vanquished, or possessed of "the rag" in response to all of life's other vicissitudes? Menstruation, like marijuana, may intensify some people's characteristics, but it doesn't usually create them. The woman who vigorously enjoys sex during her menses probably enjoys it at other times, too.

Perhaps the state of being motivated to think about something else is the best menstrual antidote of all. When women really want to attend an important meeting, write a significant paper, or meet a new lover, menstrual pain can be blocked from consciousness. Aphrodisia may even replace pain with pleasure. Being sexually infatuated or in love can diffuse almost any anguish. Whether this knack depends on a constitutional ability to produce morphinelike chemicals or whether it can be learned through harsh experience would be an interesting area for investigation.

Are women strong and sexy or sad and crazy around their menstrual time? It depends on the woman. Sometimes when it

seems that no one is doing anything for me—especially premen-
strually—I feel abandoned and sad. My patients and I know that
at these times we must be especially good to one another. When
they say, "I cried and cried last night because I kept remembering how my little dog died ten years ago," I nod with great
empathy.

My menses generally occur at the beginning of the month,
directly after bills go out. Sometimes I worry if I will get paid.
I remember my martyred grandmother who used to say, "I give
and I give and I give, and what do I get?"

My patients ask what's wrong. "I am remembering my grandmother," I tell them.

They smile with compassion and a nod of understanding.

On Fellatio

ONE OF THE amusements of being a sex therapist, besides hearing a great many bad jokes, is to run across all manner of "scholarly" comments about sex. I usually don't know whether or not they are true. In any event, they always interest me. I say to my friends, "Did you know that Cleopatra was reputed to have lowered herself [euphemism] on one hundred ten Roman legionnaires in one night?" They look fascinated and want to hear more. So I tell them that lipstick originated among ancient prostitutes who wished to announce their willingness to perform fellatio. And that Cleopatra was the best fellatrix of all, better than Josephine, or even Catherine the Great. And that it was an ancient Chinese custom for grandmothers, mothers, and nursemaids to calm little boy babies with fellatio. Also that to be a Lesbian originally meant to come from Lesbos and take penises into one's mouth, until Sappho changed all that. Fellatio, I've found, has a rich history, however apocryphal.

Fellatio is an act that reverberates to our character structure, both as givers and as receivers. We may find ourselves engaged in it for love, or lust, or a peculiar unison with someone else that transcends ordinary mating. Physically, there is nothing more to it than an exercise of oral glands and muscles upon penis, scrotum, and any other areas one cares to include, but I suspect it represents a great deal more. What we call simple, physical reality does not suffice for truth.

I have often observed that physical and psychological reality tend to be at variance. When we bathe in the ocean, we may not emerge particularly clean, compared with having had a bath, but our psyches are refreshed. When the body dies, we presume some immortal journey for the soul. So it is with fellatio, albeit a more commonplace subject. The word is derived from the Latin verb *fellare*, meaning "to suck." The activity consists of placing one's mouth on a man's penis and sucking, licking, or moving the head back and forth. Some sexual artists create a host of variations on this theme, but the basic behavior requires only the most fundamental intelligence to comprehend or accomplish. Yet the word has traversed history and linguistics to acquire extraordinarily voluminous psychological associations, considering the simplicity of the act.

I would guess that fellatio is partly a pleasureable extension of animal grooming, something like the tongue and mouth method that cats and monkeys use to clean one another. The world of sexual commerce among heterosexuals often provides it as an adjunct to bathing—at the massage parlors, for example—although the association to actual cleansing seems vestigial. Among homosexuals it is found ubiquitously in bathhouses as an unpaid service men perform for one another. Fellatio may also be related to a primitive form of identifying someone else—by smelling and tasting—as well as checking for excitability, the way male animals smell females to check them for estrus.

Another simple aspect of fellatio is that it feels very good to the men who like it—and many do prefer it to intercourse. As reason, most men cite the tight fit of the mouth as compared with a loose vagina. Pressure on the glans—especially the "deep throat" variety—is sought after, and mouths have muscles, tongues, and teeth. The various squeezing, scraping, and sucking actions that the mouth can perform far outnumber the possibilities for sensual variety inside a vagina. When one considers that hands, mouths, and bodies can be simultaneously involved in fellatio, one can see that the possibilities for sensation increase geometrically. When one also considers that a partner can administer to the entire male genital region—testicles, anus, and buttocks as well as the penis—with hands and mouth, the wonder sometimes seems to be that men like intercourse at all.

Yet people—being human and infinitely complex—have not been content to enjoy simple physical experience. They have invested fellatio with all manner of additional significance, from being an evil that must be punished vigorously to being a luxury worth fortunes. The paradoxical aspects of these attitudes call for definition because we must make our choices and live with them. Participants in fellatio had best know what act they are performing, emotionally as well as physically, both for self-protection and for achieving maximal delight.

Perhaps the most common interpretation of fellatio has been as an expression of male dominance and female submission. For some, to conquer a woman has been to spray semen onto her face or into her throat, to violate her dignity, like spitting or urinating on her. In consequence, for at least a century, many normal and self-respecting women have declined to perform fellatio.

It is important here to distinguish between fellatio and another activity called "irrumation." In fellatio, the person who sucks is in control. Irrumation, on the other hand, is the activity of the person whose member is in someone else's mouth. This may involve thrusting behavior that is clearly dominating and power-oriented. It can be painful and humiliating, unless one is constructed to withstand it, excited enough to enjoy it, or willing to use teeth, if necessary, to stop it.

In the actual practice of fellatio, not irrumation, the person practicing the act determines what is to be done. It is a totally voluntary behavior. Indeed, in times when the act was in disrepute, many women exercised it as a power to attain other goals. Being rare, it became more valuable. Like domesticated animals coming tamely after food, men often were led by their appetite for it. Even today, a woman who is highly skilled commands admiration more often than disrespect. Furthermore, men who are inadequate to perform intercourse for whatever reason may gratefully surrender to women who will satisfy them this way. And if she chooses, a woman can cause a man to feel as enslaved and unworthy as any man ever caused a woman to feel. The attitude, not the act, determines the significant effect.

On the more positive side, we may substitute the word *love* for *power* and talk of giving and taking love through this exchange. The pathways love can take through oral-genital juxtaposition are quite complex. For example, few women in my practice experience ordinary affection for their partners' members. Yet kissing a penis as though it deserved loving attention stands as a cardinal rule for good lovemaking. Rather than following technical directions for kissing, tongue flicking, and sucking in a prescribed sequence, responding naturally as an act of love, of caring for the lively, responsive organ with one's mouth, probably serves pleasure better. Treating a man's penis not only as a beloved aspect of his body but also as a unique being, like an infant or a bird, requiring the most nurturant and elegant care, is a major secret of mutual gratification.

I cannot and do not teach "erotic" behavior in the sense that Misty Beethoven, the heroine in a famous old porno movie, was taught the maneuvers of commercial sex. Yet I have had occasion to teach fellatio in its most intimate details to women whose husbands or lovers were paraplegic or suffered other disorders of mobility and decreased sensation. Such women often need to learn to become extremely vigorous with their mouths, developing really strong tongue muscles merely to be felt; they also may want to learn to overcome repugnance to using their tongues anally, for that area may retain sensitivity that the penis has lost. I have also helped women with normal husbands or partners to learn to use their mouths, if they really want to. I rarely spend any prolonged time on this, however. Once they have overcome basic inhibitions, they are usually able to learn the flourishes on their own, with help from an enthusiastic companion and a sex manual.

For most lovemaking purposes, the following fellating sequence would bring pleasure to the majority of men. It's helpful for a woman to start at a man's chest and work her way down. She can do exactly the same things to a man's breasts that he might do to hers, if he is sensitive and ample. She can hold them, suck on the nipples, circle them with her tongue, make them feel cared for. With mouth and cheeks and hair and oscillating tongue, a woman can kiss any path she pleases down past a man's navel and across his abdomen, bypassing the penis to reach the area behind his scrotum. She can move back up to his testicles, playing at them with her lips and tongue, one at a time, lightly and affectionately. A woman can really do anything she thinks of doing—tugging, pressing, kissing, licking, lapping—it doesn't much matter. It has been a fashionable wrinkle to take the testicles gently into one's mouth.

Arriving at the penis, she may want to make some preliminary greeting: a kiss, one long lick, a definite "hello." Wetting the penis very thoroughly with saliva is a good idea even though it may feel almost too wet. With one hand covering the lower half of the shaft and the other either cupping the testicles or playing at the anus, a woman may take the top half of the penis into her mouth. Playful variations include sucking on the penis, flicking the tongue around it, grazing it with teeth, twisting hand and head for a rotary flourish. She may also attempt to take the entire organ into her mouth by pretending that she is required to say "ah" for the doctor. When excitement mounts, she can curl her lips around her teeth, move her head up and down, and create vigorous suction in the best fellating tradition. The speed of stroking increases and becomes more regular as climax approaches. All this action, of course, assumes either a very well-controlled or a relatively unreactive male. A high percentage of men cannot hold back orgasm when given this much stimulation, and a woman has to be careful to stop in time, or stop frequently, if she wishes to continue on to intercourse or to extend lovemaking. A small percentage of insensitive men may require penile friction against rough clothing, a stiff washcloth, or anything else a woman can think of to elicit sensation. What may set one person reeling with pain may be only a minor stimulus to another. (Such anesthesia, however, should not go undiagnosed, especially if it is progressive.)

Just as women may need to learn to regard penises as nurturing organs, so men may be exposed to this way of thinking about themselves. Much has been made in the analytic literature of the analogy between the penis and the breast. People have tended to interpret this as a negative metaphor. For a woman to like penises too much may be a sign of excessive maternal dependence. However, there is nothing wrong with simply taking nourishment, metaphorically. For a man, the breast-penis equation may be life enhancing, too. Some men satisfy a need to give, even to be suckled, when extending their penis to a woman's mouth. The caretaking response that a man may feel for the woman at his penis could in some way relate to that during nursing.

A further paradox in thought about fellatio involves its being potentially dangerous for both men and women, while at the same time representing an act of the greatest trust.

If most men suffer castration fear, their appetite for fellatio certainly does not reflect it. They expose their penises to a veritable arsenal each time they indulge. The low rate of injury impresses one with the trust and respect that must exist between humans at the level of peacetime mating. Emergency rooms rarely treat problems of this kind, yet the potential is enormous.

Just as it is trusting for a man to place his most precious organ into that part of a woman's anatomy that can most effectively destroy it, so a woman trusts a man with her life when she takes his penis deep into her throat. Fellatio can turn suddenly to irrumation, and although death is as rare as castration or injury, it nevertheless occurs. It is more frequent between male homosexuals, but men have been known to asphyxiate their female partners too, by plugging up the larynx. At a less mortal level, there are reports in the literature of fellatio's causing petechial palate hemorrhages—destruction of small palatal blood vessels. Oral sex, therefore, can be associated with far more damage to both partners than intercourse. Performing it probably represents our human way of assuring one another that we are harmless, have good intentions, deserve trust. Just as animals often present their bottoms as a sign of deference and peaceful intention, so lovers may reassure one another that they are fangless and weapon-free, using their equipment for love and not war, by kissing and caressing one another's genitals.

There are a few men who do not like fellatio. Their partners rarely bring them to therapy because so many women are not particularly eager to perform oral sex. Occasionally women do complain of feeling rejected because their partners are not interested. The reasons for male reluctance that usually emerge (beyond simply not liking the idea) involve one form or another of castration fear—phobias of uncleanliness, fear of penis loss or damage, and so forth. Some men also fear harming their lovers. One man was afraid that he would like fellatio so much that he would no longer be in charge of his own destiny.

Often men are dissatisfied with the way their partners perform—or do not perform—the act. They may deny their dissatisfaction by saying they don't like fellatio at all. They may remain silent in aggrieved discontent. They may insist on bringing their partners to therapy to learn how, often an awkward experience for wives and therapists alike. To the man, the idea is perfectly reasonable. "Why should I go outside for it when I love my wife and want it from her?" To the woman, the whole subject seems an abuse. "Why should I be forced to do something I don't like because I'm afraid my husband will go elsewhere? It isn't fair. Why didn't he think of this before we got married?" I am not usually successful at teaching such women. The most an unwilling spouse can accomplish is a mechanical performance, which satisfies no one. And sometimes men, like women, are too shy to tell their lovers what excites them. One man had had a long-term girlfriend during his adolescence who bounced his penis dryly against her lips until he had an orgasm. He couldn't describe this to his wife without my therapeutic assistance.

Often women come to a sex therapist on their own to learn to perform fellatio. Sometimes their motives involve more than a simple desire to feel good or give pleasure to someone else. But the motives may also be inappropriate, as in the case of an insecure young woman who was willing to learn it as a degrading but necessary behavior in the search after young men. Other women ask to learn it "because my husband wants me to, but I don't want to." Rarely are such reasons acceptable. It is more important to help a woman not to feel degraded, or not to be so obedient.

More appropriate motives, beyond increasing one's own pleasure, include learning it to help stimulate a lover who needs "more" in order to achieve erection or ejaculation. A partner's impotence, or partial impotence, or tactile insensitivity may be good cause for learning new maneuvers in addition to trying other forms of sex therapy.

The more common objection women make to learning fellatio is that it is "unclean." Women do not like the idea of putting a "dirty" genital into their mouth. Often education can do little to change this. In sex, reason rarely improves passion. Nevertheless, reason states that the bacterial danger in oral sex is largely to the man. Few people appreciate how truly "dirty" mouths are, collecting all the bacteria that survive on decomposing food. Provided venereal disease is excluded as a contaminant, the people at risk of infection—developing urethritis and other disorders—are men. Yet the woman taking semen into her mouth risks AIDs more than her partner, since the concentration of virus is thought to be higher in semen than in saliva. The woman who refuses to fellate a casual partner is simply refusing to play Russian roulette. But women's reluctance, in committed relationships, is usually a way of expressing their dissatisfaction with the role of fellating, as they perceive it. Women who associate fellatio with degradation continue to feel abused by the act, and sometimes with good reason. It depends on how their partners feel about what they are doing as much as on their own attitudes.

Most prostitutes require that their partners be very clean prior to any sexual encounter, yet there are men who expect their wives or lovers to fellate them over an all-day accumulation of odor. Some women don't even know that this odor is not permanent. When they complain that "he smells," and I advise them to tell him to wash, they can be quite surprised.

Another familiar deterrent to female pleasure is the ejaculate itself. What to do with it? Certainly a woman is entitled to have a simple distaste for the smell, the consistency, or the act of receiving semen in her mouth, without any complex emotional difficulty being invoked to explain her reluctance. Some men have muskier or more rapidly developing odors and tastes than others, whose excretions are sweet and barely detectable. Another old problem is whether or not to swallow the ejaculate. It is said that men like women to swallow it as an affirmation of their manhood; conversely, women often want to reject oral contact with the ejaculate as an affirmation of their womanhood. Real battles rage on these issues, rarely soluble through any simple negotiation. Conditioning a woman to accept the ejaculate by having her practice getting used to it in stages rarely works. The reason is that couples whose only problem is disagreement over the fate of the ejaculate usually compromise. They have so much else going for them that the ejaculate does not become a pivotal issue. In those instances where the fate of the marriage seems to turn on it, the emotional as well as the sexual climate of the unit is so disturbed that whether or not a wife "swallows it" becomes a symbolic contest. One couple I know of evolved an equitable and quite interesting procedure: The woman received the ejaculate in her mouth, then shared it with the man in an open kiss; he was thrilled to take part in what was otherwise a female prerogative, and by the mutuality.

Another power struggle that may frequently arise as people engage in genital battle involves the issue of orgasmic satisfaction. Certain men—most often of low socioeconomic status, but sometimes surprisingly high on the cultural ladder—still neglect female satisfaction. Once they have been fellated to orgasm, they feel no obligation to give in return, just as some premature ejaculators feel no requirement to continue manually to satisfy their partners when they are done. Sometimes the problem is ignorance; at others it is an unconscious wish to deprive. One retarded ejaculator whom I treated was able, ultimately, to allow a woman to fellate him successfully (as long as his own hand remained at the base of his penis). But after his orgasm, he turned over and went to sleep.

I have no suggestions to offer to men who are disinclined to experience fellatio, as long as they and their partners are comfortable without it. Being kissed or fondled wherever one likes is a matter of choice, so long as it doesn't bother anyone else too much. The only generalization I can make to help men and women who experience discomfort or revulsion involves finding out why: If you like the person so much, why is it that his genital or her mouth is so unpleasant to experience? When that question is satisfactorily answered, again and always, the use of pleasurable imagery, association, and circumstance helps to blot out and cure the discomfort.

And, of course, it isn't necessary either to perform or receive fellatio "perfectly." There is no special need to be a broad-throated expert or a whip-tongued star. Whatever one likes, or feels like doing, is all there is to do. Most women use both the hands and the mouth to avoid the necessity of deep oral penetration. Some prostitutes cover their activities with a mass of hair and use only the wet hands and face for stimulation, "fooling" their customers with the motion of their heads. These are not "illegal" techniques for lovers and wives, too, so long as someone is having pleasure. However, the precaution of wearing a condom ought to be observed when appropriate, as much for fellatio as for intercourse. Casual pairing is no longer acceptable, and even "safe" sex is dangerous.

The motives for performing fellatio vary profoundly. Beyond love and erotic dominance, every nuance of intimacy may be considered, every resource of human feeling. Fellatio may constitute a convenience to eliminate contraception, a skill, an aspect of sexual variety. Perhaps too often it represents an avoidance of the closeness of sexual intercourse. Some men and women cannot merge their boundaries in coitus, others cannot bear to have sex as independently as fellatio requires. And certain men have been reported to perform fellatio on themselves in cases that involved narcissism, dependency, and power conflict—not to mention extraordinary suppleness.

Fellatio relates to love, respect, dependency, and trust. In all, it's an imperfect expression of feeling that may at best reflect our willingness to be as decent to one another as we humanly can be.

A Case of Male Sexuality

HE WAS A dramatic and erudite man. His wife, bred for pride, looked at me through the tears that had faded her high-boned face over time. He struggled briefly with the discomfort of feeling outnumbered in my office—two women and one man—and then, with some irritation, posed the great riddle.

"Men like to have sex, that's all. With a lot of women. It doesn't mean anything. Why can't my wife accept that?"

In the tales told by old masters of suspense, the statement of the mystery is often followed by a puffing of pipes and a settling down to the pleasures of a good yarn. "An interesting question," says the portly man who has until then been silent. Everyone turns to him as he exhales a stream of smoke into the turn-of-the-century night. "Let me tell you a story that to this day, to this very moment, sends a chill horror through my bones. . . ."

"An interesting question," I say to the man and his wife, who have sat before me in many incarnations. I wonder what their story is.

Many educated, cultivated men call themselves sexually "simple." Capable of grasping elaborate philosophic concepts, of creating or responding to art, music, literature, of performing mathematical feats and conceiving of other worlds, some men nevertheless insist on their sexual fundamentalism with evangelical passion. "It feels good. That's all there is to it."

What, I often ask myself, is the point of this pose of sexual simplicity?—"men like to have sex, that's all." Why should they pretend to be naïve? Why is this such a strong attitude among so many males? Is it "male sexuality"? What is "male sexuality"?

Certain men appear proud of their capacity to have erections and enjoy sexual excitement without any mental stimulation at all. The notion of an elastic, hyperactive penis may give them a sense of carefree youth. A boy's penis strains against tight clothing, bumps into tables, constantly anticipates some intriguing contact. Early sexuality may be a mindless state. Only later do emotional or psychic stimuli take on importance: a date with the "best-looking" girl; a desire to kiss a sweet young person; a wish to have an orgy; a willingness to "make love." The transition from purely physical to partly psychic excitement occurs slowly throughout childhood and adolescence; they gradually merge.

As we grow up, hormones must arrive before specifically sexual feeling can occur. When hormones arrive and a young man has no available sexual object, his sexuality may feel aggressive and perhaps detached. The hormone testosterone has been considered the key stimulus to "male" sexual behavior. To test this notion and to assess the power of testosterone, scientists have been dosing animals with it while they are still in the womb. Every mammal available to the laboratories has been found responsive to prenatal testosterone.

When a pregnant ewe is implanted with testosterone, her little female lamb will come out looking or at least acting like a male. How masculine the fetus becomes depends on the amount and timing of the hormone. Testosterone introduced early in pregnancy causes the female fetus to form masculine genitals. Later in pregnancy, it causes masculinization only of mating behavior. Testosterone even later in pregnancy masculinizes only urinating position. In normal animals, including human beings, fetal brains are programmed by this male hormone at different phases of fetal maturation to send out signals for masculine behaviors at different periods of gestation. Testosterone given to a fetus can encourage the development of male sexual organs, the soliciting of females and the mounting of them, aggression, and male urinary position in all lower mammalian life. We can surmise that it would do the same to human beings.

In any case, the messages from the testes of the normal male fetus are powerful determinants of masculinity. Normal male embryos would all remain feminine were it not for a protein called "Mullerian regression factor," which intervenes rather majestically to prevent the development of Fallopian tubes and uterus. Testosterone from the fetus then stimulates the development of male organs.

Testicles make the man as well as the fetus. They cause the male growth spurt, muscularity, deepening of the voice, sexual drive, potency, and spermatogenesis. A secretion called dihydrotestosterone causes a boy's beard and prostate to develop. According to one study, men with bass singing voices and tall heavy builds have higher testosterone levels and report greater sexual activity in the years from twenty to forty than smaller baritones and tenors. While one must be skeptical of such limited research, the fact is that up to a point the quantity of testosterone present in a male bloodstream powers the sexual engine.

We don't precisely know at what point men are hormonally

"oversexed" or "undersexed." We know what is average. We don't precisely know what is normal. We don't know exactly how sexual activity correlates with testosterone level. Some men may be driven more than others by a desire for indiscriminate mounting, female soliciting, and other sexual behaviors.

The pituitary gland controls the testes with two of the same hormones that also control female reproduction: FSH and LH. It takes about three years for the pituitary-testicular system to mature. At first the process occurs mostly at night. The pituitary releases LH in bursts during the sleep cycle. After a time, the LH effect on the testes causes testosterone to rise cyclically, too, in synchrony with REM phases. I'd suspect that this may account for an early association of male dreams with sexuality. The great cycles of manhood begin by entering the dreams and creating the image of woman in darkness.

With adulthood, LH secretion and testosterone increase during the day, as well. Six to seven short bursts of secretion usually take place during the waking hours. The highest testosterone concentration is in the morning, however, built up after the night's sleep. On the average, testosterone levels are 25 percent lower in the evening.

A man's hormonal fluctuation is such, indeed, that his very best time may be a September morning! Seasonal variations have been observed in male testosterone concentrations in the blood plasma. The lowest are in spring. They increase during summer and peak in September, according to several studies. Libido may also increase with higher concentrations. This leads one to think that starting a love affair or renewing a marriage may be most likely in the fall. (Conceiving children, however, may possibly be easiest in summer because of cyclic annual responses to light. The phenomenon of vacation pregnancy may be more a response to light than to lovemaking.)

The people who examine men most at night, these days, are

the new urologists. The era when a man in search of his sexual nature might awaken several times with an erection and reach for pen and notebook to record the dream for his psychoanalyst is now yielding to the era of the nocturnal penile tumescence monitor. The NPT monitor—among other things—studies how many full and partial erections a man has at night, when his penis is attached to strain gauges at the base and glans to measure changing circumferences. If the test takes place in a research situation, his brain waves are recorded by an electroencephalograph; his eye movements are monitored. A needle or surface electrode is placed between the base of his scrotum and his anus. We learn from these studies that male sexuality is characterized by a powerful and obvious excitement that may constantly afflict the healthy man with a desire to copulate. In one study of men in their early fifties, there was a mean of 2.4 full NPT episodes per night and 1.2 partials. In 398.8 minutes of sleep, 81.9 were spent in full erection and 24.2 were spent in partial erection. That means that a middle-aged man, even under distracting laboratory conditions, spends a quarter of his sleep-time in sexual excitement!

Male sexuality is a strenuous body activity. If men spent as much time thinking and dreaming about sex as their body spends in excitement and erections, one might wonder that copulation isn't occurring on every street corner at all times of night and day. These findings, indicating almost continuous sexual excitement, begin to help us to understand the libidinal dilemma of our dramatic and erudite hero, who came to me for absolution of his lust.

The quest after understanding male sexuality takes us into yet another laboratory. In 1979, a research team reported in *Sexual Medicine Today* that they had recorded male multiple orgasms prior to ejaculation. The graphs of heart rate, respiratory rate, and anal contractions demonstrated conclusively that orgasm and ejaculation can occur independently in normal men. The men studied, ranging in age from twenty-two to fifty-six, reported from three to ten preejaculatory orgasms per session of lovemaking. One man reported that he could, on occasion, have thirty orgasms within an hour.

Men, therefore, may not only think about sex and be driven toward it all day and night, but also are able actually to have it during much of the time. It is not just that their internal and external sexual stimulation is almost constant, if they allow themselves to be aware of it; they also may have as yet largely unexplored capacities for performance. The trick seems to be to inhibit ejaculation while going from one orgasm to the next. Although I don't recommend it, one technique is to try to urinate during orgasm. Men cannot urinate and ejaculate at the same time. If the urinary sphincter is open, the ejaculatory sphincter will be closed, and so orgasm without ejaculation may occur.

An aspect of male sexuality that has not yet much entered the laboratory is the variable detumescence period among men. Why do some sexual "athletes" retain erections for as much as half an hour after ejaculation while other men lose them instantly? Tumescence and detumescence are governed by valve-like structures (polsters or Ebner pads) containing smooth muscles that either block blood or allow it to enter the penis. When we know more about how to control these gateways, sexuality may become even more of a preoccupation among men and researchers alike.

As if hormones, night cycles, and an unexplored capacity for multiple orgasms were not enough sources of sexual unrest, nature has given men so many routes to erection, so many sources of and pathways for erotic stimuli, that the mind can hardly contain their multiplicity. Normal male function can be divided into five phases, each regulated by a different mechanism. These are libido, erection, ejaculation, orgasm, and detumescence. If I take just the first, libido, and think upon it, considering the factors that influence it, I am overwhelmed. Libido is regulated by testicular androgens. A castrate has little or no libido. Androgens can restore it. Even rats whose penises have been anesthetized with tetracaine retain their libido and continue mounting behavior. Sexual appetite and behavior continue even without genital sensation.

Libido is also regulated by what one medical text calls "poorly understood psychic factors." In this context, *regulation* is hardly the word. *Stimulation* is more like it. Very few experiences do not stimulate the libido of the apparently normal, healthy male. The feedback from all five senses, particularly vision and touch; the lure of beauty, adventure, sport, greed, dominance; the impulse to care for, protect, nourish; the desire to hurt or punish; indeed, every feeling and thought that a man may experience can lead to a heightening of the libido and a sexual response. Whether sexuality is the foundation of feelings or a relentless shadow that accompanies us, in men it affects everything.

The drive is difficult to eradicate. The ability to perform is maintained by a system with so many backups, one wonders that it isn't completely fail-safe. With so many stimuli, how do men retain their sanity?

Fortunately or unfortunately, there are a few natural downers. Because the male sexual system is so complex, more can go wrong with it. Although reproductive ability may be preserved, the act may not be quite as much fun if some of the components are missing or muted. Damaged sex can be like listening to great music on a portable radio; the grandeur may be recalled but the actual experience feels shallow and inadequate.

Apart from fear of AIDS and other sexually transmitted diseases, perhaps the greatest control of all is male vulnerability to psychic interference. The male sexual system is so immensely sensitive that a man hardly needs to know what he is thinking for the message to travel to his penis. The psychosexual disorders account for a great slowing of sexual activity. Impotence, so easy to cause, to contract, to live in fear of, keeps a sexual army at bay. The self-consciousness related to ejaculatory disturbances may deflect yet another great segment of the population from sexual sport. Finally, women, brood behavior, and aesthetics enter the picture.

In my experience, when a man does not—for whatever reason—seek to control his own sexuality, female jealousy and sensitivity take over the task. They are major deterrents, major forces that keep society more orderly than it might otherwise be. It seems to me that the male requirement for a dominant female mother figure is the most powerful, the most resented, and, paradoxically, the most sought-after control of male sexuality in our society.

Not that it works 100 percent of the time, or even 50 percent of the time. But it does seem to serve to keep males oriented to a home base. Though it forces many to lie and to conceal, they do have less sex, with less pleasure, than they might if they were free of concern about their dreadful gatekeeper, or, while single, if they weren't always searching for a woman to play the role.

Without his female bodyguard, a man might be totally subject to the wild excesses of his desire. Though he may wish to control the forces that seem to control him, often he cannot. Society does not help him to keep his life in order. And so he must invent or create a warden, a battle-ax, an infirm "old lady," a sexless, unattractive keeper of the morals, a sensitive creature whose life would be ruined if she knew, who watches for him from the window, wonders with whom he has lunch, awaits him at night, and runs his life.

I do not think that marriages deteriorate because the relationship becomes automatically incestuous and so the sex bond weakens. I think that many men unconsciously drive their marriages to this point as early as possible, in order to exert some control on the terrifying ubiquity of their sexual impulse. The old style of selecting a "good girl" served this purpose; the new style of living with a woman until it is established that she will become possessive enough to take the sexual reins serves the same end. In one case, I watched a man create a mythical guardian when his wife became entirely uninterested in his whereabouts. Perhaps when men mature and become masters of their own sexuality, as great a force to manage as that may be, we will have less marital misunderstanding. Some men do indeed take responsibility for themselves, but that is not the custom.

The major therapy for waywardness when the reins wear thin may be for a wife to refuse the role if the husband can be made to feel no shame at needing a controlling "mother." If a wife is able to overcome her own need to maintain the marriage through maternal watchfulness—if she is able to establish independence—the man will either try to seduce her into returning to the role, invent her, or train someone else to play jailer. Occasionally, he will grow up.

I cleared my throat and rearranged my feet on the small footstool I use to help keep my back straight while I am working. "An interesting question," I repeated to the dramatic, erudite man. I could envision the scenes, the tears, the hurt and withdrawal, the silent and spoken rages. At the back of my mind, the pipe-smoking English narrator was describing a scene atop an icy mountain where one man had to eat the other five frozen members of the expedition in order to survive.

My patient looked at his watch. "If this is supposed to be therapy," he said, "let's get on with it."

"Have you ever considered," I finally said after another

silence, "what feelings of distress your wife might experience at your 'sexual simplicity'?"

He reached for his wife's hand. "That's what makes it all so damn complex," he replied. "I'm a very sensitive man."

It was going to be a fascinating case.

On Ejaculation

I'M TEMPTED TO think that sex therapy often creates problems by curing problems. The thought often occurs to me when I am dealing with relationships in which the men suffer ejaculatory disturbance.

Before therapy, the main problem appears to be either quick or delayed ejaculation. The man, upset by his inability to control the flow of his semen, usually hides his feelings. The woman often expresses hers all too clearly. "We barely begin to have intercourse when suddenly it's all over. It's so frustrating and I feel so left out, I'd just as soon never have sex again." Or, "He pumps away until I'm so exhausted I want to die. I've learned to have multiple orgasms, but that doesn't mean much anymore. I'm absolutely bored and tired, totally worn out."

What is ejaculation, after all? And why does timing mean so much to women?

Ejaculation is the third of five phases of male sexual function. It consists of two processes, seminal emission and true ejaculation. Emission occurs when seminal fluid enters the urethra from the interior organs that hold and conduct sperm. Ejaculation occurs when the muscles at the base or "floor" of a man's penis contract rhythmically and the urethra expels the semen from the penis.

Both premature and retarded ejaculation may result from physical disorder. Prematurity may be caused by inflammation of the internal genital and urinary organs or the rectum. Minor irritations of nerve structures may also cause it. These, alone, may present a continual sexual stimulus and bring a man closer to the cerebral threshold for orgasm.

On the other hand, advanced damage to nerves conveying tactile stimuli from the genitals may cause local anesthesia. This can happen to women as well as to men. They may require prolonged and vigorous stimulation to compensate for loss of sensitivity. This may result in difficulty reaching, or complete inability to reach, climax.

Orgasm differs from ejaculation. In men, orgasm is psychic only. While ejaculation consists of muscle contractions and expulsion of semen, orgasm relates only to perceiving the muscle contractions as pleasant. These muscle actions may occur without any passage of sperm. If the man experiences them as pleasurable, he is having a "dry" orgasm. In any event, when a man cannot share this pleasure with a woman, she is likely to feel deprived. The premature ejaculator's partner usually feels little pleasure in his orgasm. It happens too soon for her to reach excitement or climax. It may also emerge without much contractile force, because he is trying to hold it back. The woman may not even be aware that an ejaculation has occurred, much less be stimulated by it. The retarded ejaculator who does not release inside a woman deprives her of the pleasure of his orgasm, the contractile stimulus to an orgasm of her own, and the balm of his ejaculate.

The sympathetic nervous system controls ejaculation. This same system stimulates "fight or flight" reactions to danger.

Consequently, some men ejaculate involuntarily in dangerous situations. Indeed, a great many men need to imagine strange or frightening erotic situations in order to ejaculate. This leads to considerable psychic confusion about orgasm and ejaculation, as one might imagine. On account of the peculiar way in which nature elected to use the same signal systems in our bodies for both pleasure and pain, we get all mixed up.

A man may be making love with gentle passion. His partner is sweet and tender; he is warmly loving. He strokes her hair and fondles her breasts as though she is precious to him; they rock together and kiss in a series of affectionate embraces. Slowly eroticism mounts and the lovemaking becomes vigorous, harsher, more like combat. Thrusting is strong, and the lovers may bite, scratch, or slap one another as excitement dulls their perceptions of pain. As the man approaches ejaculation, images of harming or being harmed may surge through his mind, some deviant, some simply bellicose, all generally bizarre. A particularly savage thought can trigger ejaculation. After all, the sympathetic system is in charge.

When it's over, he's confused. He wonders if he loves or hates his partner. If he's sensitive, he's ashamed of the aggression he's just experienced, and kisses softly to make up for it.

People say that if you really want to understand a man, ask for his thoughts before orgasm.

While being a human with a nervous system is better than, say, being a plant or a coelenterate, it is certainly not as refined a condition as some of us like to believe. One of the problems involves getting scared. Some men feel more anxiety than others about their sexual behavior. These ejaculate faster. Certain other men have great conflict about poorly understood hostile feelings during sex. They may ejaculate with more difficulty (although there are many other causes for delayed ejaculation, such as too much effort at planned parenthood, fear of impregnation, physical insensitivity, and so forth). One of the problems lies in having such a close neurological connection between our greatest pleasure and our warning system for pain. While masochistic and sadistic thoughts can rarely be entirely extinguished as erotic stimulants, understanding them and accepting their relationship to one's childhood can help to relieve the guilt that makes so many people's sex acts unpleasant. Although some linguists trace the root of the verb *fuck* back to the Old English *gefah,* meaning "foe," and *faege,* meaning "fated to die," I don't want to give the impression that it's necessary to have hostile thoughts to stimulate ejaculation. Many men ejaculate with eagerness, generosity, and wholesome awareness of power. They are not disturbed. Some men are triggered by destructive thoughts, however, and are troubled by them. They need help in locating the love, perhaps mangled, that lies behind the aggression.

All kinds of other thoughts may march or sidle through sexual consciousness during high excitement. Anything provoking a mild anxiety that the brain can misinterpret as pleasure will do. Beyond fantasies of being ordered to perform obsequious acts by women wearing high boots, leather gloves, and nothing else are exhibitionism, voyeurism, fetishism, homosexuality as forbidden behavior, zoophilia, pedophilia, coprophilia (feces), klismaphilia (enemas), mysophilia (filth), necrophilia (corpses), urophilia (urine)—and other delights. Some people actually act on their particular deviance, like the great sexologist Havelock Ellis, who enjoyed women urinating on his face; others are satisfied with imaginary trips to the prohibited pleasure. We are an odd lot.

Additional feelings that confuse the nervous system relate to presently occurring conflicts with a sexual partner. These may be conscious or unconscious. Conscious conflict, of course, involves any disagreement between the two lovers: whether to buy an oriental or wall-to-wall carpet; summer camp for the children versus a family vacation; the wisdom of allowing Grandma to take responsibility for the baby. A fight before bedtime, with leftover resentment, can bring on ejaculatory difficulty even in the "cured" couple.

Another related pattern for both premature and retarded ejaculators involves fear of giving love. The man who comes too quickly may be afraid of the intensity of his passion; the fear triggers the ejaculation. The man who holds back his love for fear of criticism or rejection or responsibility may also hold back his orgasm. While fear of love may lie at the root of most sexual dysfunction, we can usually treat the manifestations of the problem by working on themes involving dominance and submission, activity and passivity, giving and receiving.

Unconscious hostility may have a similar genesis in both the premature and the retarded ejaculator. They both tend to feel unduly submissive to women or else rebellious against them, largely as a result of early parental interactions. They are both usually overconcerned about pleasing a lover. One man I treated withheld his ejaculation for fear of being premature; once over the strongest urges, he could not recapture the momentum at will. He was a man who had always denied himself pleasure in order to service a sweetly tyrannical mother, and now he was trying to service his wife. He needed help in ejaculating when the impulse occurred. Until he became comfortable with enjoying sex for himself, he had to learn temporarily to disregard his partner's satisfaction.

Another man's only way of dealing with parental demands on his time and energy had been passive-aggression. If his mother asked him to do anything, it might get done, but not for a long time after she asked. By that time it would make her angry. This unconscious habit persisted through his life and made his commercial dealings difficult. It turned to disaster when he hired an attractive woman architect to design his new offices, but did not follow through by adequately describing his taste. She proceeded independently, reminding him frequently that she was worried about his time schedule and he ought to pay attention. A few weeks before the business was set to open, he observed what she had done, was dissatisfied, and demanded miracles of renovation. In sex, this same pattern caused him to withhold orgasm when he experienced the woman wanting it most, or indeed wanting it at all.

The technical "cures" for prematurity and retarded ejaculation both operate on the principle of giving control to the man. To alleviate prematurity with the "stop-start" method, the one I have accepted, the man tells his partner to stimulate him until he is near the point of orgasm but still able to hold off. He rests for ten to twenty seconds before asking her to resume. As soon as he becomes very excited again, he repeats the "stop." When he has stopped three times, he allows himself to ejaculate fully on the fourth.

In the early stages of the therapy, the man's partner uses just her hand to stimulate him. Then, when he has developed some control, she lubricates her hand with Vaseline to simulate vaginal texture. Finally, if control continues, the man graduates to the vagina itself. At first, intercourse is a rather mechanical act, though a friendly one. The man very clearly tells the woman what to do as she kneels astride him and moves back and forth on his penis, stopping and starting under his control. Later the stops and starts become so integrated into lovemaking that the man hardly has to make any conscious effort at control.

The important therapeutic task has been to remove his concern about the woman's responses. In charge, he cannot be an anxious, submissive little boy.

Treatment of retarded ejaculation involves helping the man to ejaculate when he wants to, rather than feeling he must respond to a woman's requirements. He may do this at first by masturbating while his partner remains unobtrusively still, and by ejaculating under his own control in her presence. Later, he may indicate that she is allowed to touch his stimulating hand as he ejaculates, or to receive the ejaculate on her body or in her mouth. Finally, he may choose to allow her to mount him as he ejaculates, or to continue self-stimulation to the point at which he enters her at first during and then before ejaculation. Sometimes he may have to repeat the process of stimulating himself several times until he is able to ejaculate inside the vagina. Ultimately, he may be able to begin to use a woman's vagina as though it were his hand, for his own pleasure. When he is able to do this, the sexually responsive woman's enjoyment will generally follow. Again, the therapeutic task is to remove the man's inappropriate concern about the woman's satisfaction.

An important rule in both dysfunctions is that the sufferer not masturbate for a few days before intercourse. The premature ejaculator needs to learn how to delay under conditions of some pressure. The retarded ejaculators tend to masturbate more frequently than is optimal for normal relations because it is a sex act entirely under their own control. The rule against self-stimulation has to be strict. Delayed ejaculators usually disobey it at first simply because it is a rule.

Sex therapy can even be more complex when a man suffers ejaculatory disturbance for physical reasons. Unusual personality constellations may result, imitating behavior patterns characteristic of the man whose disturbance is caused by psychological rather than physical problems. For example, a man who is premature because of chronic internal irritation may be attracted only to aloof women who do not initiate sex. With such women, he does not easily lose control. Some physically normal men may ejaculate prematurely in response to a fear of sexually aggressive or assertive women. These men, too, are likely to choose distant or unresponsive partners.

A retarded ejaculator with nerve damage may suffer humiliation when women are dissatisfied with his performance time after time, overtly or covertly. He may, therefore, find himself in multiple relations for the "safety" factor. He may develop extraordinary charisma to keep people close. He may also be able to reject them easily because he himself has been so often rejected or found wanting. He may develop an underlying hostility to women, even though it may be his nature to love and identify with them. In these cases, the psychotherapy of sexual disorder must be approached with caution because therapy based on ordinary family dynamics is not adequate to interpret the problem.

As I say, it sometimes appears that sex therapy creates problems by curing them, or attempting to cure them. The wives of premature ejaculators are often seething with repressed rage at having been deprived over so long a time. Although they agree to perform the exercise, they may become angry and reluctant when it comes time to do it. They have given so much for so long; now they are being asked to give even more in what seems to them a spiritless, mechanical way. Furthermore, if they are successful, they run the risk of losing their husbands to the wanderlust that may develop when a man wants to try out his new skill with other playmates. Suddenly treatment can seem like an exercise in further futility. Men, too, may fear alleviation as a threat to their security; they realize that they will want to experiment with others and don't want to risk knowing how to. Beyond these almost universal deterrents, the complexities of character may intervene in unpredictable ways.

Delayed ejaculators, too, may have problems with being "cured." In my practice, those whose disorder originates in hostility to women or fear of them tend to live out patterns of multiple rather than monogamous relationships, largely because they cannot tolerate any one woman exerting a singular strong influence on their life. Women also tend to leave them after the first thrills of orgasm or multiple orgasm wear off and weariness sets in. If the man is courteous or intelligent enough not to exhaust his partners, they may depart anyway, from feeling inadequate to elicit sexual release and from the pressures of being otherwise dominated or left "wanting more." If these men gain sexual control, they are deprived of an important "repetition compulsion," which they have used to frustrate female satisfaction. More direct aggression may threaten to surface.

Those exceptional relationships where retarded ejaculators remain monogamously loyal before and after "cure" offer at once the most vocal power struggles that I encounter in my work and the scenes of tenderest reconciliation. Suddenly these men, experiencing themselves as fully in charge, are not sure whether to behave as dictators or helpless children. Instead of being passive-aggressive, they are passive one moment and aggressive the next. They drive their wives and their psychiatrists crazy for a while.

It is, of course, inaccurate to say that by curing problems, sex therapy creates problems—but it does reveal them. For many, true therapy begins only after the sexual disorder has cleared. The problem, I've come to realize, becomes a question of purpose. For example, in the case of curing prematurity, what does lasting longer accomplish? Being able to have sex for an extended period of time may help a woman to have orgasm and improve the intensity of the man's ejaculation. Beyond that, making sex last does not improve the *quality* of love or lovemaking. Nor does abbreviating a sex act that tends to run overtime do more than shorten an onerous task, unless something more significant than having an orgasm is going on. At this point, if not long before, the techniques of sex therapy only serve to demonstrate the importance of old values. Ultimately, the dilemma is: What for?

The Orgasmic Revolution

NOT LONG AGO, I treated a woman whose mother had told her repeatedly of the joys of breast-feeding and the horrors of intercourse with brutal men. As a result she was unable to have a genital orgasm but could climax if her breasts were stimulated. She did not know it, but that woman was a heroine of the orgasmic revolution.

In counterrevolt against the supremacy of the male-dominated "vaginal" orgasm, women recently began to defend their sensations. Early researchers had found that all orgasms have a common path. The same muscles and blood vessels were said to be involved in the same contractions, no matter where on her body a woman is stimulated. The first revolutionary banners, therefore, proclaimed liberation from the need to have orgasm with a male organ inside. A woman could be emotionally mature even if she had orgasm "only" on clitoral stimulation. It was the same orgasm that she had when stimulated anywhere else.

I remember the political change from the seeking of total "fusion" with a man to becoming "independent." More than one woman sought sexual help because she was unable to masturbate alone or respond to her lover's tongue and fingers instead of just his penis. These women were often able to climax only on intercourse. Many were able to reach orgasm only after being triggered by their lovers' ejaculations. In spite of what might have been described as perfect sex by the generation that saw simultaneous orgasms as ideal, these women were truly disturbed by their dependence on men. One woman felt that if she could have her own orgasm, she could go out and get her own job, which was precisely what she did after learning how to climax by herself.

The revolution went even further. Women began to develop a kind of reverse discrimination by honoring the sensuality of the person who could achieve orgasm easily by means other than direct genital contact. "Clitoral" orgasm was deemed excellent, but women who had orgasm by breast and nipple stimulation formed the varsity of sexual achievers, to be topped only by those who had orgasm on fantasy alone. By these standards, the frightened and constricted woman who came to me to be treated because only her breasts were sensitive, while her genitals were numb, was a sexual champion, a freedom leader.

By now we should be largely educated to the philosophy of not discriminating against a woman because of the site of the sexual stimulation that encourages her to orgasm. She is welcome to have any sort of climax she pleases, without any imputations about her psychosexual maturity. Considering the vast turmoil in their patients' lives, psychiatrists have hardly the time or inclination to pass out edicts about the proper stimulus points for sexual pleasure.

We reserve the right to a few qualifications, however. Although healers used to take the "vaginal" orgasm too seriously, it is still reasonable for women to enjoy heterosexual intercourse and respond to it with orgasm. The concept of orgasmic equality was a fine revolutionary credo, but being able to have orgasm during coitus remains an acceptable pleasure, one to be sought. Even though some noncoitally orgasmic women display more independence and other fine qualities than some women who have coital orgasm, I think they are still missing something. I sense that a percentage of these women who cannot truly enjoy intercourse do have problems in intimate relating. They may have difficulty in communicating simple sexual desires; they may be unable to assert themselves; they may be victims of deep-rooted and persistent conflict. There is usually some psychological problem, however small or large, when a woman fails to climax with modest frequency during sex with a competent and likable lover.

Now that the first rush of independence is over, the sexual scholars are taking a second look. Freud has been revisited and found not so inhumane. All he said was that to enjoy intercourse fully one had to shift the erotic focus from the clitoris to the vagina. That seems at least partly true as long as clitoral sensitivity is retained. Considering that we have been revering orgasm produced by thought, or a kiss on the eyelids, we can hardly object to the mental or physical pleasure that encourages a woman to climax because she likes the idea and feeling that her vagina has a secure hold on a penis.

I have my doubts about the creed of orgasmic equality and its insistence that climaxes achieved by any method of stimulation, from sweaty penises to bejeweled vibrators, are all the same. I don't mean to suggest that orgasm experienced by oneself with the aid of a feather, Coke bottle, or oscillating toothbrush, or astride an electric shoe buffer is any the less an orgasm. There would seem to be some question about the emotional satisfaction one may achieve from these objects, however. Devotion from a Duracell battery can hardly be compared to male adoration. Is it too much to say that under most circumstances the latter seems preferable?

Admittedly, not every orgasm achieved through intercourse is marvelous. One woman tells me of having small and lonely orgasms while her lover, mounted from behind, kneels and pumps mechanically. Another describes the empty, routine "quickies" with which her partner services her, ejaculating within seconds of entry. He is able to delay if he wants to, but since she is capable of rapid orgasm, he sees no point in doing so. A third woman describes the ritual she must fulfill in order to excite her lover: She must play the part of a stranger, or observer, or some fantasy role that dissociates her from her own warm feelings. He becomes powerfully excited if she creates a particularly convincing scene and then makes love to her with his full muscular penis as no other man ever has. Yet the aftermath always leaves her sad and empty, in spite of dozens of orgasms.

Could any of these three women be blamed for occasionally wishing she could skip the next desolate coupling and have a healthy session with a vibrator under her own control?

An orgasm is an orgasm; a rose is always a rose. But some are more beautiful than others, and some gardens surpass all human design.

On Sex and Pregnancy

LATELY, PREGNANCY AS a sexually heightened time has gained much publicity. The prophets of the new sexuality include sex during pregnancy as one of the wonders we do not sufficiently know. A woman big with child, they tell us, can enjoy sex with enlarged gusto. Pregnancy is described as a highly erotic experience for those who can abandon old fears.

Perhaps so. I doubt it. Perhaps my own experience and that of women who seek help from me are skewed to the darker side. To me, pregnancy is not sexual paradise. Maybe it would be paradisiacal if nothing else were going on. Usually, however, other things are happening both within a woman's psyche and in the outside world.

In the world outside her body, the ordinary devastations of everyday life may be proceeding at a hectic pace: A woman's other children may be suffering their usual quotient of childhood plagues. Her own siblings may be disturbed and causing competitive friction. Her parents may be distracted by their own troubles, or simply on a trip around the world when they are most needed. The crumbling of the family unit in our society is reflected not merely by divorce statistics. Women are now often left on their own to raise their progeny with washing machines and microwave ovens instead of Grandma. In many ways, it's easier. In others, the price is high. I wonder whether or not the incidence of postpartum depression and suicide among young mothers will increase because of this sharp decline in the traditional sources of concern, no matter how much they may be resented by "independent" young women.

A woman's husband may also be reacting to pressures. Now that he potentially has "another mouth to feed"—a responsibility that he often feels acutely, even if no special desperation is necessary—he wants to increase his income. He works harder, thereby isolating himself from the family. Frequently, he takes solace in another woman, perhaps someone with whom he works. Or if he is not the sort to seek sexual consolation, he becomes deeply involved in his work or his hobby. A man may resent, however unconsciously, the attention a pregnant woman may get from family or friends, and this may also lead to male withdrawal—or competition. None of this is very easy on the woman.

In the first trimester, a long pilgrimage of concerns may file through her mind. An important decision must be made at the outset: whether to keep the child or to have an abortion. Pregnancies are not always voluntary, and besides, few educated women enter motherhood absolutely wholeheartedly in this curious time. Does the world need another human being to add to the glut that may drive us to destroy ourselves completely? Can one really afford a child? Even when a baby is wanted, many women spend the first few weeks in doubt about whether to hold on to it. The magnitude of the decision often leads to strained sexual relations. The pressures are so intense—the physiological, psychological, and social changes so dramatic—that I sometimes feel that the miracle of early pregnancy is how few acute psychoses develop at this time. One must designate this period as a time of primary stress. Perhaps only the elevated hormone levels protect women from madness.

Once the pregnancy has been accepted, a woman often takes a semi-invalid stance. She may become more sexually passive, if she is interested at all. Sometimes, "morning sickness" keeps her from feeling entirely well. If the couple makes love at all, the act may be tenuous and exploratory—he gently finding out what she will tolerate, making love as though she were ill; she preoccupied with providing for the baby's comfort and care.

During the second trimester, the simple increase in fetal size seems to discourage many from sex. A woman who was never secure with her self-image (too fat, too disproportionate) may find herself becoming profoundly altered for the worse, and feel even more inadequate. Too often, also, women lose what physical fitness they possess during this period. They neglect to exercise and they overeat capriciously. Sexuality decreases even further.

As the last trimester begins, the child is very obviously present. Soon it is profoundly in the way. The baby literally gets between the parents. It seems determined to separate the couple, physically as well as emotionally, protruding between husband and wife. They may unite, but not closely. And so yet another change must occur in the style and passions of the young couple. On the physical level, they must learn to adjust positions, abandoning the male superior for a while. This can present difficulties, because many couples simply have never experimented beyond the missionary approach, and many women cannot make sexual requests. Even among more versatile lovers, the loss of closeness can be quite real in those who require total frontal contact, chest to chest and belly to belly, for feelings of security and completeness.

Sex therapists are frequently called upon to advise regarding positions. The most commonly taught is the T, in which the woman lies on her back, her head on the pillows. The man lies at a right angle to her, his body under her legs. He may insert his penis sideways, from underneath her thighs. Side-to-side positions can also be arranged. Most often the woman puts one leg under the lover's waist and both lie on their sides, facing each other slightly. A woman may straddle her lover, if she and the baby are comfortable. Or intercourse may be had from behind, or in any other position gymnastically feasible.

The psychosexual realignment of the last trimester is far more complex than the physical. These later months involve a struggle with gross frontal mass, even if all goes well. Clumsiness can be so disheartening that many women are convinced that their husbands are too polite to tell their true feelings. And indeed, some men do perform only to make their wives feel wanted. The husband's sex drive may in fact decline as the wife's pregnancy becomes more apparent. Men tend to suffer in silence with their fears of castration, of damaging the fetus, of being poor fathers, and of soiling their wives, who have now become "madonnas."

Women worry too. They wonder what their organs will be like after the emerging bulk of the infant has pressed its way through the vagina. They observe their stretch marks. They contemplate the slack that will occur in their breast tissue when they are done with nursing. Their nipples will be brown instead of the original pink. They know that their visual sex appeal will inevitably be less to men brought up in a youth culture—and even to themselves. We tend to see ourselves as others see us.

Women who have recently had children often feel jealous of all the svelte young creatures parading about, and sometimes they let it ruin their marriages. Experiences in the singles world behind them and with statistics freely available, most know that their husband is likely to find, or be tempted to find, another partner at the same time that their child is on the way.

Women wonder, too, whether they are going to be adequate mothers. They question whether they'll have enough patience or delight in motherhood to do the job. Today's standard for child raising demands a psychological sophistication that few women feel they possess.

More couples than ever are coming to me for sex therapy during pregnancy. They usually arrive at my office in the second trimester. Things haven't been going well sexually; they want to make them better "before the baby is born" because "after that, it will be too late." One of my most interesting recent cases was that of a fifty-five-year-old female banking executive in Chicago, married for fifteen years to a man twelve years her junior. An adoption agency was about to give the couple a child, to be delivered in three months. She arranged to take a month's vacation in New York so that she could see me. "I want to have orgasms on intercourse before I have the child," she explained. Why? "I want my husband to feel closer to me before the baby comes. I don't want him to feel rejected," she said. Since her problem related only indirectly to orgasm, I set the goal of therapy as working out ways to reduce his potential feelings of rejection and her fears of abandonment. Six months after the baby was delivered, when all three were functioning happily together, she spent two more weeks with me and was able to free her orgasm from psychological constraint.

Another group of intriguing cases, which reflect the new mores, involve women who have their first affairs during pregnancy. Given that the fertilized state may be a source of considerable psychological distress, a turn-off, a time of major agitation, why should women turn to extramarital relations?

Again, sex can work as a defense against depressed feelings, even for the impregnated.

Some women, too, "know" that their husbands are now wandering, even without open discussion. They now need a man's support through the birth of their child and often turn seriously to someone else. Male doctors—pediatricians, obstetricians—often find themselves in intensely caring and sexual roles during these times, though on the surface it might seem a violation of medical ethics to have such relations. The men who deliver women and help them most to care for their children afterward often become the recipients of a love that transcends the patient-professional relationship. Sometimes I treat the woman who has given her love to such a man, and who often gives him up when the crisis subsides. And sometimes I find myself treating the devastated male physician, whose professional demands have so demolished his private life that all he can have are these fleeting periods of engagement with needy patients.

Experience suggests that the abundant sensual ecstasies of pregnancy are, for many of us, a product of the mythmakers' dreams. Statistics presented at the World Congress of Sexology in 1979, pertaining to Italy, Germany, and Denmark, indicated that sexuality as measured by intercourse frequency and subjective sensations of desire declined in linear fashion throughout pregnancy. Recent American studies agree with this finding, although one study by Masters and Johnson back in 1966 showed increased desire in the second trimester. On the whole, however, according to reserved findings, as they grow larger with child, women want sex less.

But warmhearted people can gentle a new life into being while making honest love to one another during the entire nine months of gestation. Ideally, we have the impulse to tend life, to husband it, to make it thrive. The child symbolizes our union, and orgasms can swell around it. The baby becomes consciously incorporated into the sex act. The man strokes his wife and the substantial outline of the child with the same tenderness. It seems possible that the baby experiences all this with some pleasure. Certainly the rhythms of rocking in infancy resemble the pleasant jostle of coitus. As for the woman, she begins to respond both as herself and as herself-with-child. No longer is she the sole recipient of her lover's attentions. She and the baby very clearly must share.

Perhaps nature contrived the long duration of human pregnancy to give people a chance to learn to love their offspring as they love themselves and to give the necessary and appropriate erotic dimension to the loving of a child. Natural caretakers do not question the ultimate existence of the child or their own ability to nurture it. They love, they create, they work.

That's the ideal. For a lucky few, that's how pregnancy is. For others, I know it can be that way at least part of the time. The realities of existence are often severe, but people and other animals go on birthing, foaling, dropping, whelping, and calving in an enormous propagative travail. We must know both pain and pleasure. Properly appreciated, they can make that first furious scream a sound not only of birth but also of resurrection.

On Sex and Nursing

In THE 1950s, when I had my first baby, the idea that nursing could be an erotic experience would have raised eyebrows.

Nursing was enjoying a revival in the fifties. "Formula" was no longer universally regarded as an ingenious modern improvement upon the ancient method, a means of preserving a mother's energy. Although the medical reasons were obscure to us, the new mothers of my generation felt that the close body contact of nursing must be good for children psychologically. Those of us who could, did. For people who liked privacy as much as I always have, nursing seemed to offer the opportunity to be left alone—to recuperate from childbirth, regain strength, and gradually renew our interest in sex.

For people who did not like solitude, however, nursing was a lonely time of commitment to an uncertain ideal. Perhaps it induced security in the child, but it was not so psychologically wonderful for the mother. Nursing separated the mother from society. The baby was not company; it still felt like a part of oneself.

As I nursed my baby in the 1950s, I became aware of certain physical feelings that reports were only beginning to detail in the 1980s when this book was first conceived. Studies indicated that many women experienced heightened breast or genital sensitivity within four to six weeks postpartum. I felt this increased sexual awareness, yet I had no desire to have intercourse for several more months. As I now know, nature actively contrives to reduce sexual behavior during nursing by supplying less estrogen. Often the nursing mother does not lubricate easily. The vaginal walls may thin out. Sex can hurt. Members of a symposium in the journal called *The Female Patient* noted that this is particularly true of the woman who is pregnant for the first time.

Yet the nursing mother cannot avoid focusing on her erotic organs. She is often stimulated by her baby and ashamed of that excitement. It seems wrong and abnormal, somehow, to have excitement—even a dry, unlubricated orgasm—while nursing an innocent infant. Will the child develop an Oedipal complex? If the husband enters the room while the orgasm is occurring, will he accept that there is really no wish to translate the fleeting erotic experience with the baby to intercourse with him? After all the obstetrical cutting and sewing, the sitting on inflated tubes, and what with the nursing bras, the flabby midline, and especially the odor of warm milk continually emanating from one's chest, the notion of performing the act that began all this travail may seem a bit too much. Sexual feelings when nursing a baby can be a reflex response. One may wish not to have it, but like the male erection, it occurs.

Even though some women may have no trouble declining intercourse after childbirth, many are also under pressure to reaffirm—to themselves and their mates—that they still can perform as sexual partners. They may also have a strong need to be held and comforted. Since many men are unable to be tender, women learn to make sex substitute for comforting. Thus, even soon after childbirth, they often seek sexual union though their body may not be ready for it.

For all these reasons, a nursing mother may agree to intercourse. Her breasts may not want fondling. Foreplay can be uncomfortable. It may seem as if sex will be difficult for a long time to come. If the new mother and her husband do not know about her low estrogen levels, he may feel intensely rejected and she may wonder what is going on in her psyche.

Tradition, while it had the fault of isolating women, mandated respect for their need for peace and privacy. Women nursed alone, or among women friends or attendants. Polite and educated men did not expect sexual return from a woman in the throes of producing milk and giving her body to her child. They might find someone else to satisfy their lust, but they were not supposed to intrude upon the nursing chamber, nor was it considered good form to press their desires in the bedroom.

Young people, today as always, pay more attention to their ideals than to their feelings. Women, seeking liberation from any social exclusion or sexist privilege, attempt to carry on life with baby as without it. To prove they are not weakened by being women, they will be as sexual and erotic as they ever were. In doing so they fall into another sexist trap: the myth that women can and should desire sexual relations at any time of the day or month. When they do not, men tend to consider this withdrawal as a neurotic symptom. But medical research indicates that women experience cycles of lust. If they do not feel erotic during the nursing period, that is the normal response.

The notion that sex should be more fun during nursing might seem to gain authority from the biological observation that fertility decreases at this time. Without much risk of another pregnancy, some say, one ought to be able to cavort at will. This, of course, is yet another utilitarian bias. Many women, when they are not easily fertile, feel less rather than more amorous. One cannot conclude that the nursing period ought to be a time for sexual marathon simply because children will not be born of it.

As things generally work out, even with ideas about high sexuality during nursing, couples do not often slip into free and glorious congress, enhanced by the sweetness of milk and the infant's plump contentment. More frequently, they come to realize that this is a temporary hiatus in their sexual pleasures and try to avoid a cycle of hurt and rejection.

Some authorities advocate that women use lubricants amply during this period. If the new mother is lively and emotionally invested in sex, lubricants may be welcome. If she is not, she has reason to hope that nature will calm down her husband. New research indicates that male hormones respond to female patterns, although as yet only a monthly, cyclic response has been demonstrated; husband as well as wife, therefore, may undergo a temporary abatement of high erotic interest. If the waiting period becomes prolonged and intolerable, it may be that a power struggle of another sort is going on. A sensible doctor may suggest a switch to formula and a vacation, without baby, on a warm, sensual island, but we need to be alert to the potential for any failure of sexuality to signify deeper conflicts.

Not long after I'd brought my first baby home from the hospital, my doctor paid a house call. I had a cold; I was feverish and underweight. I'd been nursing the baby, coping with the practical nurse, and wondering when my episiotomy would heal. We stood next to the crib where my dumpling-cheeked son was sleeping. "That's one fat baby," the doctor said. He pinched my arm through my robe and showed me that no flesh would stay between his fingers. "Too thin," he said, shaking his head. "Too thin."

"So?" I asked.

He said, "Stop nursing."

Though it was physically painful and emotionally trying, I did what he told me to do. My time alone with the baby was gone. Other people could feed my son. The special bond between us was broken. I think I would have survived being "too thin" for a while.

Today, very little doubt exists about the advisability, even the necessity, of breast-feeding in spite of concerns about toxic environmental contents. We are sure that breast milk contains many substances important to the baby's health. The immunoglobulins, for example, protect children against various diseases. The psychological benefits to mother and child are also no longer disputed. To avoid loneliness, young mothers, as part of the sexual revolution of the sixties, began to nurse their children at parties, in restaurants, at work. It is no longer surprising when a hostess at a dinner party opens her blouse and offers her full breast to a passionately ingesting little mouth.

Nursing may be peaceful and joyous in the presence of one's husband, as well. Not all women suffer estrogen depletion—or even enough hormonal variation to cause significant physical deficits—and many couples include their nursing infant as a member of the primal scene. While feeding progresses, some women can engage in foreplay and gentle intercourse. For them this provides a unique delight and may be a means of deflecting the father's natural jealousy.

Nursing plays a role in relation to love and tenderness, as well as to jealousy and abandonment. Women's capacity to nurse is, paradoxically, as necessary a part of human sexuality as it is a deterrent. One obvious factor relates to men's appreciation of suckling and caressing breasts; another less often discussed aspect is the woman's response.

Psychologically, nursing usually coincides in women with a strong caretaking urge. The contractions of childbirth are associated with the release of the hormone oxytocin, which stimulates milk letdown. A mother's response to this hormone is to engage in active mothering. But childbirth is not the only time this can happen. When a woman who has not recently given birth is suckled, made love to, or has an orgasm with uterine contractions, her milk letdown reflex may be stimulated, just as it is in childbirth and nursing. Some women actually secrete breast milk during orgasm; photographs have been taken of the droplets emerging from one such woman's nipples. In this respect, having an orgasm rather resembles having a baby.

Along with milk letdown, intercourse and particularly orgasm also may stimulate the caretaking response in a woman who is not a new mother; but the feelings she would have had for the baby are transferred to her lover. These emotions subtly help to bond a sexually adequate marriage. They also are at the heart of another of those astounding and little-known differences between men and women. On the morning after a particularly intense sexual experience, a woman may be driven, however irrationally, by feelings that impel her to nest her lover as though he is a new infant. During subsequent days, she may wish to buy presents, make meals, or take care in whatever way she knows. This drive has vast implications concerning the desolation so many women feel after short trysts or vacation romances. The popular belief that a woman who suffers this way is too much governed by her own dependency needs may be ill-founded. Her anguish may also arise from having lost someone whom her body, often in conflict with her intellect, recognizes as a helpless creature who depends on her.

On Impotence

"NO, WE ARE not trained to ask routinely about people's sex lives," the third-year medical student said as we sat in our white coats and discussed patients in 1980. "Wouldn't it be embarrassing?" he asked. "I mean, I can't imagine talking so personally."

I had begun to feel something more than frustration. After the decades that my colleagues and I had spent advancing the concept that sexual dysfunction could be an important symptom of physical illness, it had not yet become a routine area for questioning patients at the large New York hospital where I taught sexual psychology. Students were taught to ask about everything else—headache, vision, hearing, appetite, digestion, chest pain, arm pain, back pain, breathing. They inquired about the color, consistency, and frequency of bowel movements and the urgency of urination, but questions about erection, ejaculation, and orgasm were not "part of the printed sheet." Nor were questions regularly asked about any function of the female reproductive tract except menstruation. It may have been some measure of modern medicine that prostatitis was discovered more often by asking about urinary irregularities than by inquiry into

113

the symptom of pain on ejaculation. Indeed, one of the most complete textbooks of internal medicine at the time did not even mention ejaculatory pain as a possible symptom of that disorder!

Sex therapists rather than elder physicians were left to inspire students to respect the sex organs not only as procreative tools and the toys of love, but also as indicators of sickness. It is said that "sex is not a matter of life and death." Yet I saw no greater link to the process of living and dying than sexuality. At the minimum, it seemed to me that doctors ought to ask about all forms of sexual discomfort. A woman who complained of pain on intercourse might have anything from herpes to cancer. A man experiencing impotence might suffer anything from diabetes to multiple sclerosis. Still the students did not ask, "Do you have erections?" "Do you have any pain or problems related to these activities?" People too quickly assumed that all such discomfort or trouble was psychological.

Medicine was not the only field to have ignored sexual disorder—and to have ignored impotence in particular. With rare exceptions, serious literature gave it short shrift. Writers were far more enterprising in exploring the lust of Lady Chatterley's lover than they were in considering the dilemma of Lady Chatterley's husband. Even after Jake Barnes, the emasculated hero of Ernest Hemingway's novel *The Sun Also Rises*, the American storyteller's preoccupation with sex consistently presumed good function. Such failure of awareness has been a romantic tradition—not unlike the prescribed design of a morality play— that limited perceptions of the diversity of human character as reflected in our sexuality as well as our theology.

On the other side of the medical establishment, researchers and a growing cadre of physicians enthusiastically accepted the sex organs as a scholarly concern of medicine and came forward almost daily with new studies, new relationships of function to disease, new drug effects. The days when a man would go to his doctor and confess his problem only to be told, "Relax and you'll be fine," were soon to be over. Physicians would not be so quick to refer impotent men to psychiatrists, either, until they had taken a proper history and done the necessary studies. One of the tactical problems of my practice was to return a patient to his physician (or to suggest a specialist) for the multiple tests involved in proper diagnosis. A myth had been perpetrated that 90 percent of impotence was psychogenic—in the mind. Among my patients—people who were often already screened by other physicians—the figure was more like 60 percent psychogenic as far as I could tell at the time. I guessed that only about one-third of the impotence suffered was entirely psychological in origin.

Today, in 1994, I'm told that explicit questions about sexuality are still not asked by many doctors, but enough attention is paid so that only about 20 percent of the patients who come to me for potency problems have simple psychogenic impotence, a dysfunction caused by conscious or unconscious anger or alarm. The rest suffer a major or a minor physical impairment. Sometimes erections are not quite full. Even though they are sufficient to penetrate, a man may be self-conscious about using them. I can help by advising him how to achieve his best erections without psychological interference.

Diagnostic techniques have advanced sufficiently that sexual awareness is more commonplace among urologists, even if many other doctors still lack sexological confidence. Some urologists refer patients to me most often, these days, to assist them to become psychologically accustomed to their sexual aids, like injection therapy or the vacuum pump. In an aging population, men increasingly are being taught to inject a few drops of liquid under their penile skin to allow their blood vessels to expand so that blood can come in to fill the penis to a long-lasting erection, although FDA approval for this process has been slow in coming. Sometimes they need help in being less intimidated by this method. Occasionally, their wives need help in understanding that it is not their fault—not their lack of attractiveness—that causes their husbands to need chemical assistance. The same is true of the use of the vacuum pump—a device that creates a vacuum around the penis so that blood will flow in to fill it. People need help in ways that are too various to describe to become accustomed to a plastic accompaniment to their lovemaking. Nevertheless, when they do accept these aids, they often describe their relations as better than ever.

Some new aids that are being developed include a suppository a man can place inside his urethra that will take the place of an injection. Topical creams and sprays may also be of some benefit, although researchers feel the suppositories will be more effective. Whatever assistance modern medicine will be able to give to the joys of intercourse, some people will need help in accepting any intrusion.

Twenty years ago, it was considered medically sophisticated to recognize that not only diabetes, but latent diabetes—the kind that only shows up as an abnormal curve on an extended glucose tolerance test—could be associated with impotence. Now we know that approximately half the men who develop diabetes will have symptoms of impotence in the first six years. The list of possibilities for disorder has grown longer and longer. Today, the penis as a barometer of disease, present or approaching, has gained significant respect. Its erection may be affected by vascular, endocrine, drug, neurologic, and local causes. It is one of the most sensitive and responsive organs in the body.

Variations in erectile quality may lead to detection or confirmation of heart or blood vessel disease. Any time the heart cannot pump strongly enough to send blood racing through the body, the penis may not rise so easily. It requires a great rushing of blood to the pelvic area, a strong heart, and open, flexible blood vessels to produce a firm erection. High blood pressure, arteriosclerotic disease, aortic problems, coronary artery disease, disorders of heart rhythm, and lung disorders that affect the heart, like emphysema, can interfere with rapid and easy filling of the penis.

Impotence may also signal derangement in the chemistry that makes men feel masculine, assertive, and strong. Lack of sex hormones, particularly testosterone, can cause loss of erection, but the days of giving all men who suffer impotence a trial course of testosterone injections are—or should be—over. Too many serious illnesses may prevent testosterone production. For example, a brain tumor can interfere with the production of those hormones that stimulate the testes to make testosterone. One should have appropriate imaging studies to be sure no masses are pressing on the pituitary gland.

A substance in the bloodstream that may cause impotence by interfering with testosterone production is prolactin. Too much prolactin can cause too little testosterone. One may need to use special drugs to reduce prolactin.

Too much or too little thyroid hormone production may also cause impotence. A man may need replacement or reduction of his thyroid hormone.

Neurological disease affects erections. The spinal cord or sacral nerve roots may have suffered damage from a tumor, a protruding intervertebral disk, or multiple sclerosis. Parkinsonism and anterior temporal lobe epilepsy have been associated with impotence. Perhaps most fascinating of all, the polyneuropathies (symmetrical destruction of sensory nerve fibers) may lead to impotence by progressively decreasing touch sensitivity. Alcohol, vitamin B deficiency, and diabetes are some causes of polyneuropathy. Syphilis and disease of the dorsal (sensory) spinal root ganglia are others.

Most obviously, direct damage to the genitourinary and rectal areas may harm the nerves and cause impotence. These nerves may be deliberately—or occasionally accidentally—cut in operations such as radical prostatectomy for cancer, bladder surgery, removal of the testes, hernia repair, and aortic bypass surgery. Dozens of other congenital and heritable diseases, adrenal abnormalities, anemias, genital malformations, and disorders such as Peyronie's disease can lead to impotence.

The number of prescription and nonprescription drugs that are known to have an effect on the human nervous system, blood vessels, and hormones has increased at an extraordinarily rapid rate over the past decade. This is the largest category in the list of causes of impotence in current textbooks, although drug effects were barely recognized in the '70s. If you are taking *any drug at all*, it's important—if you are having erectile trouble—to ask your physician whether it affects potency. While many drugs do not, the number that do would be too great to enumerate here. The most common categories are antiandrogens, antihypertensives, anticholinergics, antidepressants, antipsychotics, sedative and anti-anxiety drugs, and recreational and addictive drugs like alcohol, tobacco, and heroin.

Ruling out or excluding the organic as a source of impotence is not a simple procedure to be accomplished by a look and a poke. The tests are diverse and have grown quite numerous since this book was first written. Physicians still do screening evaluations of nightly erections with the nocturnal penile tumescence test, to which a rigidity measuring device may now be added. These are a guide to function and are not intended as diagnostic. Penile blood pressure or "pulse volume" may be compared with pressure in the arm. Some doctors measure penile response to erotic films shown in their office rather than sending expensive instruments home with their patients. Sonography of various kinds can detect superficial penile arterial pressure, direction of bloodflow, diameter and thickness of arterial walls, and the difference between arteries and veins.

More invasively, injections of a variety of substances into the penis cause erections that could not occur if blood flow were blocked. Arteriography (X-ray visualization with contrast medium) can then detect obstructions. If blood can't get through the artery, you can see the blockage on X-ray. Beyond arterial problems, filling the penis with a special solution can detect leakage from the veins as a possible cause of difficulty sustaining erections. Drainage may also be visualized on X-ray.

Neurological testing of erections is not diagnostic but helps to exclude many diseases. Reflexes, sensitivity to vibration, and the rate at which urine flows are non-invasive tests. Responses to electrical stimulation are semi-invasive and may locate lesions in the spine. Measurement of spontaneous electrical activity may also explore the penile nervous system more specifically.

No matter how much testing is done, however, an overall clinical assessment—what the doctor thinks after he or she has talked to the patient—is considered the single most important approach.

The physician should order routine blood tests, urinalysis, and measures of blood lipids and serum components. To become more specific, plasma testosterone (total, free, and biologically active), LH, and the thyroid indicators may be measured. Urinary steroids, free cortisol, and total urinary testosterone may need to be studied. Diabetes should be thoroughly evaluated and plasma prolactin measured. The person suffering impotence shouldn't be surprised by the extent and expense of a proper work-up. Unfortunately, doctors who are meticulous in their considerations of other body systems may still occasionally feel no urgency about a thorough sexual examination.

Once the sex therapist is fairly sure the cause of impotence is not physical, he or she can turn to the mind. The therapist needs first to distinguish between the impotence of depression and other forms of disorder, such as the impotence of anxiety, or the impotence of hostility. When a man is truly depressed, he neither sleeps nor eats well, nor does he enjoy any work or recreation. His sex drive and erectile ability may disappear entirely, without regard for partner or circumstance. The impotence of true depression may be as completely debilitating as that caused by any organic damage. Fortunately, it is reversible when the depression lifts.

Other forms of psychogenic impotence really consist of erectile failure in particular situations or circumstances, as compared to physical impotence, which occurs at all times. If potency is defined as the ability to have and maintain a strong erection, then true impotence constitutes an inability to do this whether masturbating, awakening in the morning, or trying to make love. Situational or circumstantial impotence means that a strong erection occurs in one circumstance but not another. It may be primary—as in the male virgin who can have erections but not intercourse—or secondary, in men who have lost the ability for satisfactory erections on intercourse. Usually men have morning erections or can masturbate easily, but lose their hardness on attempting coitus. The reasons for this loss and the "cure" for it are the stuff of sex therapy—after the therapist is sure that nothing physical is seriously wrong. Most often, however, impotence is partially physical and partly psychogenic; perhaps my most important role is to help men achieve the best possible function in spite of disability. A diabetic man was making love with semi-hard erections, for example, but when he found out that diabetes was associated with impotence, he feared losing his erectile ability entirely, and so lost it through fear. I helped him to regain his former ability. Often I try to help people with partial deficits to make the best use of what they do have.

The "official" preliminary treatment for impotence, known as "sensate focus," is simplistic to the point of absurdity, yet it remains a core technique for what has been known as sex therapy. By itself, I would guess it to be only a little more useful than the advice that local therapists like Grandpa and the grocer might have given in the old days, although occasionally it works without any need for additional information or treatment. As a probe, however, a suggested behavior that one can use to see what happens and go on from there, it is invaluable. Around it, a sexual psychotherapy may be built. What I say to a couple when I suggest it includes the following instructions, over a period of several weeks:

The man and the woman are to take turns stroking each other as gently and lovingly as they know how. First the woman lies on her belly and allows the man to stroke her from the top of her head down to the soles of her feet; he is to touch areas like the back of her neck and the soft space behind her knees that he might not normally reach. The stroking is light, soft, and slow, neither massaging nor patting, just sensual and affectionate. After about ten minutes, she turns over and he strokes her face, neck, shoulders, arms, and on down, avoiding genital areas. After another ten minutes or so, she does the same to him.

If a man can have an erection, he usually does so under these circumstances, but he is told he is not to "use" it no matter how excited he becomes. (Sometimes he "disobeys," and his impotence is alleviated for the moment.) If the couple responds positively and obediently to the sensate focus that includes the genitals, they may go on to "nondemand" intercourse, in which the woman slowly helps the man to become accustomed to having an erection inside her without feeling the need to satisfy her or please her. She mounts him and moves gently back and forth on his penis without attempting to bring him or herself to orgasm. Ultimately they complete the full sequence of foreplay, mounting and thrusting, and climax.

Rarely, however, do these instructions do more than open a path to the revelation of what is really wrong either with a partner or a relationship. Often men are totally unable to convey their affection by stroking; they are too awkward, they have no patience, they can't learn how. They may not even understand affection—or sensuality—at all. Or women can't receive sensual gratification; it is too luxurious, too ticklish, too boring. They feel like a piece of meat being salted, or they would rather get on with their housework. Or communication doesn't work: a man loves to have his belly stroked; she keeps kneading his arms. Whatever the discord, it usually leads to discovery of the more unconscious conflicts about sex, affection, dominance, submission, appearance, intellectual pursuit, sensual relaxation, and all the rest. Frequently, one simply stops the behavioral approach at this point and starts to deal with either intrapsychic or interpersonal problems as they are reflected in the ability to stroke or be stroked. What emerges in the dialogues that follow may be called psychosexual therapy or the psychotherapy of sexual disorder. Eventually, it may or may not become necessary to return to sensate focus. Some of the time, it is not. People may ultimately select and enjoy their own forms of sexual expression, which are occasionally far removed from the balmy softness of nondemand pleasuring.

Understanding of sexual neurology in the '70s added further dimension to techniques that a sex therapist might employ and to the directions that sexual psychotherapy could take. For instance, work with men whose sacral spinal cords had been damaged showed that they might still get erections through thinking exciting thoughts or seeing, hearing, or smelling erotic stimuli.

Even though their penile touch pathways—the nerves that run from the skin of their penis to the bottom of the spinal cord, up to the brain, and back to the erectile organs—could no longer function because the brain was cut off from perceiving touch, they could still "think up" an erection, or get one in response to visual, auditory, or olfactory input. Their brain could send messages down the sides of the spinal cord, out through the bottom thoracic and the top lumbar vertebrae, to the erectile organs. A man so afflicted would not have any feelings when his penile skin was touched. But he could look down and see that his erection was there. He could use it to make love, though his only pleasure would be in the mental imagery. That is why some men with minor impairments of their touch systems, perhaps from lower spinal trauma, need more visual stimulation and mental imagery than others to enjoy sex.

Therefore, sex therapists began to encourage patients to understand, accept, perhaps alter, and eventually use their fantasies for excitement. Sometimes they had to learn to fantasize as a new experience. The past required exploration. The present needed change. The future had to be trusted. Whether or not to encourage patients to go beyond exciting fantasy and role playing into "kinky" thought and behavior for the sake of potency was a dilemma. Personally, I did not encourage it. Indeed, when a patient seemed entirely dependent on deviant stimuli for erection, I wanted to be sure to rule out epilepsy or other damage to the brain.

Yet, I did—and do try—within reasonable bounds, to assist those impotent men (and physically damaged women, too) who are not able to respond to touch and the more pastoral passions. They may need to be freed to experience exciting thoughts, to distract them from performance fears as well as to arouse them. These thoughts are sometimes not genteel and law-abiding. I am told everyone knows that when a boy steals a comic book or drives over the speed limit, he often gets an erection. This is antisocial behavior, but as an occasional indulgence it seems within normal limits. The man who must fantasize significant violence to attain arousal needs help in understanding his fantasy more than anything else.

Another path to erection is "reflexogenic," or automatic, without involvement of the brain. It has not been mapped with absolute precision. Even when no messages reach a man's head, no sense of touch, no smell, no sight of any exquisite female body, no breath of any sigh, erections may still occur through a nervous pathway—involving touch stimulation—that does not include the brain. Nature preserves man's reproductive ability with great tenacity. Even if a man's spinal cord is injured above the level where messages from his mind may reach his penis, a boomerang-type route—from, say, skin to spinal cord and back to erectile bodies—may still operate. If men had to proceed through life like the three proverbial monkeys who let no information in, they could still have a copulatory tool.

The most common psychotherapy of impotence relates to solving conflict in men's power relations with women, as the name of the disorder suggests. There may be a very direct relationship between male impotence and being weak with women. Even in these days of the woman, as always, many men have to be assertive to preserve their sexual dignity. The relaxation technique may help resolve this conflict. On the one hand, it instructs the man to be passive. On the other hand, it instructs him to expect gratification. He must not be enslaved by a compulsion to please his partner. This freedom from oversolicitousness and this instruction to feel entitled to pleasure are frequently sexually exciting.

Sometimes the passive–assertive mode is not enough, and a man requires help in being actively assertive. He needs to do as he pleases with his partner, or to tell her what to do. The requests he may learn to make are occasionally as simple and physical as, "Please move your elbow; it's in my ribs." Sometimes they are more complex: "I would like you to stop asking me to put the house in your name because I don't intend to." When a man learns to express his strength, he often feels a pleasurable excitement—the kind of stimulation that seems to me a neglected area in "conventional" sex therapy.

There are relationships between an impotent man and a woman in which active rejecting behavior is more to the point than attempts at relaxation. I'm thinking particularly of the poor fellow attempting coitus with a partner who is always either a hostile victim or an aggressive opponent.

The woman who is a hostile victim always suffers and inflicts guilt. Her partner's flaccid penis is an insult, a direct assault on her self-esteem, causing her to feel massively inadequate. He must do something about her condition instantly! The aggressive opponent considers a flaccid penis an instrument of war, an organ to be battled. She curses it in rage and calls it unspeakable names. It is proof of her lover's hatred, his evil character, the underlying sickness of his soul. She wants to know what masochism in her drives her to accept his money and his services despite it.

Obviously in these two instances, impotence is a healthy response to a partner's character disorder. The man needs to be potent enough only to rise from the bed and take his lady into the living room for a talk, or to the nearest therapist, or back to her apartment or her mother. Relaxation, sensate focus, and nondemand pleasuring are destined to fail.

Is there, I ask myself, a contradiction between the importance of sexual assertiveness and the vast need of our male population to learn to be affectionate? In practice—in bed—there is not. We have passed through eras admiring sexual aggression and through more recent times idealizing sexual solicitude. The new truth seems to be that excitement and moderate mastery are vital to sexual response. I would guess that most good lovers, male and female, consider that an old truth.

The study and treatment of impotence emphasize the enormous relationship between mind and body, the intricate connections of the brain to every organ, and particularly to the sex organs. They point up the danger of separating physical and mental problems. Those unskilled in psychology may leave impotent men to founder on the shoals of a failed "technique" or inconclusive medical tests, and those who know psychology but not physiology may waste untold numbers of therapeutic hours. In trusting others to know the proper tests, one should choose a physician specializing in sexual dysfunction; for treatment, one should also carefully choose a psychiatrist or psychologist experienced in handling the mental mechanisms—and able as well to make evaluation of the meaning and completeness of the tests administered. Perhaps one may not find precisely the right blend of sympathetic and parasympathetic stimulation, activity and passivity, masculinity and femininity, strength and malleability, decisiveness and open-mindedness, reason and compassion, or aggression and love in oneself, a mate, or a therapist. It is important, however, that all of us have some inkling of what we are looking for.

Interlude:
On Fantasy

A PATIENT OF mine relives a favorite fantasy at least twice a week at bedtime. She is a busy lawyer with little time for extended relaxation. In the fantasy, a distinguished man visits her as a potential client. He tells her his legal problem. As he talks, the sound of his voice attracts her. She especially enjoys the way he puts words together. She also finds his looks so appealing that what he is saying recedes into the background. Suddenly, they are no longer talking in her office but are sitting side by side on a banquette at a restaurant in France. He is kissing her unreservedly in public while the headwaiter beams and other couples look on enviously. Soon they are making love, somewhere in Japan, in a cool, dim, matted room where one candle is burning. As the candle slowly burns down and flickers out, she falls asleep.

Another patient tells me his bedtime fantasy. As he is sitting on a park bench one surreal day in autumn, a black uniformed woman rides up to him on a motorcycle. She signals him to ride on the back seat. He climbs on. She takes him to a large gray prison where he is placed alone in the center of a concrete room. Four uniformed women direct him to undress and to masturbate. His erection grows as they watch him impassively. Finally, he obeys them and begins to stroke himself. Each time he approaches climax, they begin to laugh and he cannot release his orgasm. He must continue to masturbate, stopping each time they laugh. Finally he conceals his excitement, and they do not observe that he is close. He quietly has his climax. They whip him for cheating them of the pleasure of delaying him. Exhausted, he contentedly falls asleep.

It seems clear to me that these two fantasies belong to different genres. One is a romance in which a woman wishes to escape the daily restraints of her profession and behave impulsively. The other is a ritual act of masochism constructed by a man with power conflicts about women. Obviously this man and this woman would not find each other's fantasies exciting. One person's exhilarating sexual daydream may be another's nightmare. The sentiment that causes one human being to snigger may bring another to orgasm. People's tastes in fantasy differ so vastly that all a sex therapist can do is accept the fantasy, and try to find the real meaning. Most fantasies have at least a dual significance. Finding the hidden significance in a fantasy, especially one that is disturbing to a patient, may be the most therapeutic act one can perform. For example, fantasies are often wish fulfillments. That seems simple enough. The complexity lies in locating the wish that is fulfilled.

An older patient, impotent for physical reasons, described a fantasy of watching his beautiful young wife make love to the attractive young carpenter who had been repairing their home. Occasionally he could achieve partial erection with this fantasy.

He brought his concern about the fantasy to me because he was troubled by the specter of homosexuality. He felt it was "queer as hell" to enjoy imagining another man making love to his wife. Perhaps there was homoerotic pleasure at viewing the imagined scene. From another viewpoint, however, the "second man" is often what the dreamer wishes himself to be, in this case young and potent. Many men with sexual dysfunctions routinely require a "second man" in their fantasies to do for the woman what they themselves cannot do: have strong erections, sustain intercourse, ejaculate easily. Sometimes the requirement for another man becomes not only a part of fantasy but also a part of real life. One premature ejaculator, a perennial bachelor, could not feel sexual affection for a woman until he was certain that her orgasmic needs were satisfied by her husband's penis. Until he was secure in that, he felt he carried too much of the responsibility for satisfying her. When women wanted to leave their husbands for him, he rejected them and sought out new partners. He, wondered, too, if he was really homosexual. One might argue that the homoerotic fantasy causes the dysfunction rather than results from it. However, I have seen such fantasy emerge in men whose lives had been otherwise untroubled by guilt about same-sex relations. The fantasies occurred *after* an episode of impotence and after the onset of ejaculatory disturbance.

Women, too, may replace themselves in fantasy by more beautiful people, or pretend their lovers are pleased by someone else's responsiveness. Insecurity is a large source of pseudo-homosexual fantasy and behavior.

In another type of fantasy, people often imagine themselves loved by long sequences or large groups of people and feel ashamed of their "exhibitionism" or their "greed." While there are many underlying reasons for such fantasy, one of the most common is failure to have been accepted as an attractive male or female by one's parents. Endless reaffirmation of attractiveness by countless men or women, in fantasy as in life, may become necessary. Like the movie star who needs to see herself in a production to know she exists, the person with basic insecurity about being found lovable or sexually attractive may require a stream of admirers. One young woman whose father seduced not only a wide variety of women but also many of her friends found herself following his erotic example. Her father had never told her that he found her attractive, or even lovable for other than sexual qualities. He rarely gave her affection. Indeed, he stayed away from her deliberately because he was afraid of being tempted to seek erotic gratification with her. Everyone could "have," could sexually possess, my patient's father except her. The multiple lovers she came to require were all, in a sense, her unattainable parent.

In fantasy or in life, many men who make love to a lot of women (or women who must make love to many men, singly or in groups) are often looking for the unequivocal care, appreciation, and love that they did not earlier receive and that would have been a foundation for the strength to be alone, or to love more singularly. They may spend their days moving from one "good mother" to the next. Like Pooh bear, they may stop all day at an assortment of honey jars, to be caressed and made love to. This seems innocent enough, although it can be complicated. One man I treated spent his time among five women: his wife, his lover, his mistress in another city, his marital counselor (whom he seduced), and his secretary. He also had relations with a series of female clients. The problem was that he always became violently dissatisfied by the quality of the women's affection, usually after proving himself totally benign and lovable. He then had to move on to conquer again the old failure with his inadequate parent.

I don't present these fantasies as the reason all men or women desire "seconds" or multiple partners, but merely to show that our mental (and physical) lives often fulfill wishes of which we may not be aware.

"Curing" people's fantasy lives is a delicate matter. The idea smacks of precisely the kind of mind-mechanics that have always made me wary. Yet if most problems are psychic, what else to do but try to alter the psyche?

The problem in therapy is twofold: helping a person to understand why he or she has the trouble, and then assisting change. Helping people to understand has been the classic activity of psychotherapy since it began. Actively intervening to help a person get better is relatively new, sparked by behavior therapy. What I have had to struggle with is not elucidating dynamics so much as inventing ways to promote change at the fundamental erotic level.

How does one stimulate a person to have sexual fantasy without being a part of the fantasy? How does one change an already existing and exciting fantasy if it offends the patient's sensibilities? And how far should a feminist therapist go in the crusade against pornography as sexual fantasy when patients might need the naughty stimulus?

I have little personal interest in commercial pornography, although I appreciate visual erotica and sensuality in art. There is a considerable difference between *Deep Throat* and the long bare line of Nefertiti's neck. If my idealism had not been enough to turn me away from the exploitive attitudes, my medical and surgical education would have reduced the novel impact of hard-core close-ups. I think this is especially true for me because I went to medical school in an era when men hazed women students. On my first day among the corpses in anatomy lab, the tips of twelve preserved penises, stuck with colored toothpicks, were brought to me on a plate. Throughout my career on the wards, I seemed to get the bulk of the genital and fecal work—

the catheterizations, the collection of stool specimens on a gloved finger. In the operating room, surgeons enjoyed directing me in the performance of certain procedures—the removal of Coca-Cola bottles and other items from the rectums of anally erotic folk; adult circumcisions; total penectomies whenever they came up on the schedule. I really know what penises, testicles, vaginas, and anuses look like. I don't need Technicolor.

Consequently, when a woman who has difficulty becoming excited comes to me to develop her fantasy life in order to feel erotic, I do not send her to the latest porno show or in search of the most recent fantasies by Nancy Friday. Perhaps the blood would rush to her loins faster if she read for the first time about having a penis in every orifice, or fantasized having her vagina exposed on midnight television. However, I feel a responsibility about training a woman's mind. The naïve woman, unexposed to pornography, often becomes aroused by that which degrades her by appealing to her greatest insecurities. Many therapists liberally recommend these stimuli without realizing how they abuse female self-esteem. I cannot prescribe pornography except as a probe, a small, well-understood step in a woman's continued sexual awakening.

One of the techniques I use to shape a woman's sexuality is to search for what has given her pleasure in the past. Many women who do not experience joy in sex do not experience much ecstasy in the rest of their life, either. Yet there is usually something in the variety of other activities and relationships that brings them satisfaction. Over time, and through conditioning, I try to help women associate their aesthetic pleasures and their simple physical enjoyments with making love, on the theory that if a pleasure—the enjoyment of a painting or music, or of merely lying on a beach—is recollected during sex, it will eventually be associated with the act without in any way degrading my patients. Eroticism grows from pleasure.

To do sex therapy without endorsing pornography while at the same time not being doctrinaire when it is useful or necessary has been difficult. People whose sex lives are governed by it, who cannot feel aroused by any other imagery, have come to that barren place through deprivation. They have little enough. It is not for me to take it away.

Many women come to me nowadays to "cure" their masochistic fantasies. They enjoy sex while dreaming of being abused. Personally and politically they are humiliated by their fantasies. Can I help? Usually I can, in some way, although we don't always succeed in eradicating the fantasy. Society used to instill female masochism through its restrictiveness, and the idea of being forced to have sex so that one doesn't have to take responsibility for the decision is too appealing to most women over thirty for them to give it up.

First my patients must understand that they truly don't want to be abused. Perhaps they wish to please another person by giving him or her a sense of power. Maybe they will get love this way, as they got attention from a cruel parent. Maybe they are punishing themselves—for hostility, for disobedience, for being born women. Once we know why, change can begin. Yet sexual masochism clings tenaciously to many women, even after everything else has been done: achieving economic self-sufficiency, developing the ability to blame others more than oneself, asserting one's desires, rights, and needs. Even if self-destructive imagery won't leave, at least reality can be better. Fortunately, the mark of the masochist is not indelible. Many women can achieve pleasure without suffering.

Men, too, bring me problems with their masochistic fantasies. The man whose bedtime fantasy I related was a retarded ejaculator with an obvious dominance problem. The "female police" were always in charge. They were punitive, enjoyed his discomfort, and denied him joy. Nevertheless, he held on to them. It was a long time before he could learn to give pleasure fully to himself or others.

Sadistic fantasy, too, troubles people enough to come to therapy, and in my practice it is far more prevalent in men than in women. The presenting complaint is usually retarded or premature ejaculation. Perhaps the most common syndrome belongs to the men who cannot ejaculate unless they have violent thoughts. Consequently, their orgasms rarely feel good, since—unlike true sadists—they have not accepted the enjoyment of violence.

Many of these men have had mothers who were excessively involved with them—by being too helpless, too seductive, too overprotective, or too demanding. The physical bond to mother becomes sexualized but is experienced as repugnant; feelings of love and attachment are markedly ambivalent. Such men may fear vigorous thrusting because the accompanying violent fantasy is too painful. One patient could not accept his thoughts of splitting the woman in half; another feared the wish that the explosion of his ejaculation would shatter his partner's abdomen. Understanding that the violence is intended to destroy the mother's power, not the partner's body, often helps.

In one way or another, a huge population of men and women suffers from hostile overattachment to mother, but the symptom of ejaculatory disturbance, interference with the life-affirming act of sexual release, is particularly difficult. When a man is so fearful that he ejaculates rapidly or tries so hard to contain his violence that he does not ejaculate at all inside a woman, it may seem to him—as it does, indeed, to us—that the very best part of his life is missing.

Fantasy, then, enters every aspect of sexual therapy, from helping women to become excited or have orgasms, to distracting impotent men from their performance anxiety, to dealing with the complex forces that govern male pleasure. Certain physical conditions, too, like impairment of genital sensation for any organic reason, such as diabetes or spinal injury, may be compensated to some extent by training in fantasy as well as by increased stimulation.

In my personal and clinical experience, some form of fantasy seems a requirement for pleasure in lovemaking. When couples don't enjoy one another, they have probably lost the fantasy that brought them together, or they never had one in the first place.

Fantasy, as a psychiatrist understands it, includes far more than the creation of "scenes," those mental pictures of sex acts that are like cartoons and caricatures of human passions. Fantasy involves any mental activity about sex, including any aura from current reading or entertainment that people may bring to bed with them, any vision of security or adventure that inspires lovemaking, or any idealization that one person makes of another. Fantasy not only relates to memories of reality past, but to memories of fantasies long since dead. The people with whom one has made love may visit again to enhance or destroy present passion; the people with whom one may wish to make love extend themselves seductively or require intriguing pursuit. Sometimes the fantasy of a goal achieved may be temporarily sated by sleeping with someone who has achieved it; at other times, too, we may imagine that we become like the person with whom we have sex. The uses of fantasy are complex and generally more positive than negative; the situation I am called upon most often to repair is the fractured dream.

I find this the real challenge of therapy. Beyond the self-punishment, sadism, voyeurism, and exhibitionism that shape certain mental pleasures, and beyond dreams of pulchritudinous grandeur, I perceive with admiration the honest aspirations that make people feel as though they want to make love with one another for a lifetime. These larger fantasies that we have about one another are at once the most fragile, mysterious, and durable of our assets. When they fail, it is urgently important to find out why.

On Midlife
Sexuality

MY MOTHER IS both the toughest woman in the East and the least depressed person I have ever met. I always wondered at the source of her aggressive good spirits.

Soon after my father died, in the spring of 1972, she received a letter from her first and only love. He was a scholar and a poet, and had been a professor at the theological seminary where she had become certified to teach history, Hebrew, Bible, and religion. At the height of her passion, he had left my mother to recover from tuberculosis in Israel. He had never returned, and she had never followed him. Now he was writing to ask if she had a "villa" for him to use if he should come to America to collate his manuscripts and ready the body of his work for the archives.

Did she have a villa? She had a hotel, a resort, constructed with the tireless dedication of an empire builder. Within its gaudy shell she had already created a private apartment: an improbable, scholarly retreat furnished with a down-filled antique French couch, a man's writing desk, and an armoire fitted out for files and storage. Had she been preparing for him? She wrote to offer it.

Of course, he never came to America. Cancer.

They correspond still, long letters on airmail paper. He tells my mother how much he loves her writing and asks why she gave herself up to commerce. They have decided it is better that she does not travel to see him. The disappointment at seeing each other now might be too great. Her hair used to be bright red, while his was soft and black.

My mother continues, happier and tougher than ever. She has never complained of an ache or pain. She fights endless battles in the conduct of her business. She has never asked for help from anyone. I recently asked her if she remembered going through menopause. Indeed, she did. Was it painful? Had she become sad? "I don't know," she answered. "I never notice my body. I don't have time to think of such things."

People can pass through menopause without a quaver, as my mother's experience testifies. Some of us have stronger characters or a greater capacity for enduring fantasy than others. But what about those of us who cannot come to terms so easily with the life and death of our dreams when we pass through menopause or climacteric?

Testosterone levels in many men begin to decline after forty or fifty, but a substantial decrease may not begin until after seventy. Men retain their ability to produce sperm indefinitely. Male erectile and ejaculatory ability tends to diminish, too. Men often need to have more stimulation to gain an erection. They have longer "refractory times" between erections and are able to ejaculate less frequently. It is important, however, not to expect these deficits as an inevitable consequence of middle age.

Small arterial occlusions (blockages of arteries to the penis) may interfere with penile blood flow. The prostatic enlargement that occurs in 80 to 85 percent of men over fifty may interfere with ejaculatory ease or force. Age in itself does not reduce the ability to function sexually. One must attempt to trace the cause. The penis is an organ, like an eye or an ear. Just as we seek glasses or hearing aids, so we may attend to improving sexual facility.

Menopause, from the Greek words signifying the end of the monthly cycles, gives women a sharp signal that the end is soon to come. Bleeding ceases. We cannot have babies. A large part of ourselves—our ovarian function—literally dies. The medical evidence that signifies this death appears in our estrogen levels; they fall, though not necessarily dramatically, for nature tries to replace what she has taken away. A woman's adrenal gland begins to secrete more of a weaker hormone, estrone, to sustain function.

Nevertheless, a woman's vagina may dry gradually because of depleted estrogen after menopause. She may need hormone replacement, orally or topically, to alleviate this condition. The argument about replacement estrogen causing an increased incidence of breast or intrauterine cancer appears to be resolving in the direction of decrease rather than increase among women who have taken estrogen along with periodic progesterone for birth control. Questions about progesterone, progestins and breast cancer have not been entirely resolved, but the hormones continue to be recommended, soon possibly in micronized form to preserve the cardiac benefits of estrogen. Our recent insight into the genetics of breast cancer may improve predictability.

Other physical manifestations of menopause include the poorly understood "hot flashes" as well as varying degrees of trouble with the menses themselves. Estrogens help alleviate hot flashes: the Menopausal Unit at the Boston Hospital for

Women did an early study that suggested oral medroxyprogesterone as a possible source of relief. Other hormones are continually being tried experimentally. Scanty, irregular, or excessive menses are often dealt with through the appropriate use of progesterone.

For a woman, the most difficult problem may be loss of reproductive ability. She responds according to personality. Some women mourn. Some become angry. Some deny they have any feeling at all. A woman's reactions to becoming sterile also depend on what fertility has meant to her. Has she had children? As many as she wanted? Too many? Did she have pain or despair related to abortion or miscarriage? Have any of her children died? How did she feel during pregnancy? Was she never able to become pregnant? Has birth control been a problem?

Loss of the ability to have children is by no means universally mourned. It may be a great relief, to some people. In one important study, only 10 percent of women regretted the cessation of their menses. On the other hand, there are women who feel right only during pregnancy, and women whose lives seem barren without an infant in the nursery. For them, often mothers a dozen times over, the end is not the relief it might seem.

The previous deaths of unborn or living children may make menopause a sad occasion. Women who have lost offspring feel grief not so much for the termination of their fertility as for their dead children. Hot flashes resemble the sweat of grieving; in the early morning, when the heat under blankets collects, a wet forehead, neck, and shoulders can feel like the flush of helpless rage when we know that someone has permanently gone. Indeed, the entire roster of other losses may unroll before we face the day; sometimes a depression is precipitated.

Menstrual loss seems to forebode the end of sexuality, too. Most women are accustomed to cyclic fluctuations of desire, based on our menses. Whether we enjoy sex most during the flow, in the period after, or during the moments before, over time we have come to develop a pattern that is part of our lives; now we fear it will disappear.

Nature lets women down gently. Among only 8 percent do the menses stop abruptly. The rest may either have varying periods in a pattern of declining frequency. We become accustomed to less. There is time to adjust to the new pattern and to become pleased with longer intervals without discomfort. "Shadow" menses occur, too, contractions without expulsion. The same cyclic feelings may persist until they gradually disappear. If we do not focus on the trouble, it may not be so dramatic.

Much of what we anticipate depends on what we have experienced. How one's mother responded to menopause may govern what one expects for oneself. My mother ignored her climacteric. It is likely I shall attempt to imitate her. Paying no attention may be difficult, however, for I am more invested in sexual reality and less in fantasy than my mother is.

Men, too, respond to their mates' changes by taking example from the past, and particularly from their fathers. If their fathers were understanding, they are likely to be too. Yet husbands who have spent a lifetime of sexual closeness, aware of every nuance of change in their wives' bodies, may ignore this momentous event. Traditionally, men detach from the fertility issue; it is not theirs. They don't talk about it to their friends. There are men, however, who identify with the loss just as other men experience birth pain. They, too, feel depleted and infertile. Many men cope with the menopause by buying their wives the best present they can afford when they become certain of what is happening.

I am fascinated with the ways men and women treat midlife as related to money and work. For men, the slide into middle age can be the best or the worst of times. All that a man has built may pyramid to pleasure. Conversely, stress and sexual insecurity may combine to propel men to impulsive behavior. They may desert their wives, indulge in abortive affairs, or destroy their families. They may change professions or life-styles in ways that seem to offer no advantage.

Women, I find, more frequently alter the distance between home and the "world" during midlife. Sometimes a woman begins to go to school or to work. Or she may retire from an active life to her garden and kitchen. We do not, however, hear much about major career changes, like beginning a new company on the other side of the country. The "home-versus-office" dichotomy usually provides enough of a spectrum.

Do women tend to be depressed at this time? We used to believe that melancholy and menopause comprised a syndrome. A recent study, however, has shown that women, particularly poor ones, who tend to blame themselves rather than others, suffer more depression than any other group including menopausal women. Another broad study indicates that the symptoms long described as menopausal—insomnia, irritability, feeling "down"—do not affect menopausal women significantly more than they do others. The word *menopause* no longer has specific psychological connotations.

At medical school, we studied a disease called "involutional melancholia." We memorized its characteristics: anxiety, worry, agitation, insomnia, feelings of guilt, and "somatic preoccupation"—concern with the idea that one's body is going to seed or becoming diseased. Perhaps antidepressant medication has reduced the frequency of this disorder. On the psychiatric service in hospitals we observed these symptoms frequently. Now depressive symptoms in women seem to decrease gradually after age thirty-five, although many of the women with depressive histories tend to have recurrence of their anxious states.

Life dilemmas cluster between age forty and sixty. All our defenses—denial, isolation, indifference, self-sacrifice, aggression—rally to meet the emotional strain. A person's sexuality, too, becomes intimately related to the struggle for a new and vital peace.

Just as we must face separating from our parents in adolescence, so in midlife the major crisis that most of us face is the final separation from our parents—death. A consequence of our first separation from home may be to discover another person with whom to share our lives. So we may be moved to find others when our parents die. When the still figure under the white seersucker coverlet of the hospital bed is buried, we go on and attempt to fill our emptiness.

Often we are not rational about our need. We grow angry at the dead: They have deserted us. We grow angry at the living: They do not care for us as they should. Our wives or husbands seem enmeshed in their own trivial preoccupations, or they have long since withdrawn their emotional support. We are often vulnerable to the first person who responds to our loss. He or she may become the recipient of a lifetime's wish to love and to be loved. Sometimes we choose wisely. We may marry, if we have not been married before, or divorce and remarry, when separation by death stirs us to further separation in life. Sometimes the remarriage is more figurative. People who maintain marriages that do not serve a comforting purpose may make long-term sexual commitments outside their legal confines in the clandestine beds of mourning. These unions may be especially strong if both partners come to them in grief.

We may bond, then, sexually as we may never have before—without considerations of finance, childbearing, and all the other factors that dilute erotic ecstasy. We may make our last pacts with life and death and the devil.

We may attain this new love and sexuality if we are fortunate. Certainly, we are just as lucky if our old supports hold, and our mates or lovers provide eager comfort, but that seems rare—at least in the world that it is given a psychiatrist to see. We may also be unfortunate and find only a transient emotional or sexual liaison that, like a chocolate with a poison center, affords pleasure rich but brief, leaving us to experience a dual loss. The world may punish us, as the people we have selected to replace the dead desert us. Or we may try to punish the world for our wound by raging through a series of people whom we discover to be only shards of humanity, hardly worthy of the ejaculate we have given them or the orgasm that briefly pulsated around their member.

In midlife, in our fifties, we are frequently lost in time. Our spirits and our bodies often seem at disparate purposes, seeking rest and resolution at the same time as excitement and rebirth. We wonder if our love is better for being ripe; or is it aging, inelastic, unable to recuperate from defeats? Sexuality resonates with separation in the intricate polyphony of our middle years, when the music is supposed to be "mature." We listen for the full development of the theme, but sometimes we cannot even make out the statement.

There are other separations, too, much less definitive than death, that are supposed, even, to be joyful. Our children sometimes take so much of our love with them as they go away to school, to work, to marry, that we can feel that they have left none behind. Longer lives and earlier marriages make the "empty nest" a space that couples may expect to share for a very long time. Children's departures may cause a greater sense of loss than most people can imagine before it happens.

With whom do we replace our children? Men often have a special love for young women at this time. Is it their own youth that they wish returned, or do they also seek replacement of their daughters? Does a daughter's parting free the incestuous bond? Or are fathers competing, like comrades, with their sons?

Women have lately loved young men more openly, too, often after their own sons have left for school or work or marriage.

Perhaps we develop a sense of how many close people we need to have about us for our family structures, and seek always to keep that alignment: father and mother figures, sibling replacements, surrogate children. Strong sexual feelings may substitute for the intensities of family bonds.

The statistics show that extramarital sex increases in later decades. They seem to indicate that older people become "freer" sexually. Perhaps that is true. But I would judge, from my practice, that the rise actually reflects people's greater losses as they age and their greater need for intimate bonding.

Nymphomania Reconsidered

MANY WOMEN WHO came to me during the sexual revolution shared a remarkable premise: they felt entitled to enjoy sex as often as they wanted it, with whomever they liked. Most of these women were unmarried, but a few of the married ones also required explicit sexual freedom. It had not always been so. Time was when any woman who behaved in that manner was stigmatized. The scarlet letter was on her breast; men exchanged her name; she was handed about like a quoit in a ring toss game. She acquired the notorious label of *nymphomaniac*.

Understanding the female nymphomaniac became a psychiatric preoccupation many years ago, as the profession scrambled to comprehend the new, sexually aggressive woman. A well-known study came up with a finding that was reassuring to alarmed males. Women, it was asserted, were not having sex for the pleasure of it so much as to be held by a man, to be warmed and nurtured. Nymphomania was explained as a desire for emotional succor through sex. Professionals were pleased with this finding; it was consistent with their view of the difference between male and female temperaments.

I suspect that few sex therapists today are satisfied with that as a total explanation for the hypersexual trend among women. Women may like to be held more than men do, but this does not tell us why they like to have sex more often than was once considered the norm. Nor, to anybody who has treated one, does it describe the real nymphomaniac.

The truest nymphomaniac is the woman in the manic phase of manic-depressive psychosis. I would guess the term really derives from her behavior. She is overtalkative, often to the point of making no sense. She may spend far more money than she has. She may be involved in a hundred new projects, or merely moving through an unproductive life like a whirlwind. Her desire for sex may be continual; she may make active advances to whoever happens to be nearby. In the psychiatric hospital, controlling such a patient's sexuality is a difficult task. These patients often copulate with the male manic-depressives anywhere they can find a space—in the halls, bedrooms, bathrooms. Some hospitals once followed a policy of discharging them for breaking sexual rules; more recently the behavior has been treated as a nonpunishable part of the illness.

Nonpsychotic nymphomania involves similar behavior. It is an addiction, in fact, that blots out feelings such as the desire to be held. A major characteristic, as described in *Medical Aspects of Human Sexuality,* is an ungovernable need to have coitus, with or without pleasure. The term also connotes degradation: a woman so driven that any male organ, hung from whatever unworthy torso, will do. Finally, it denotes an inability ever to be emotionally or physically satiated.

I have treated only one patient who approached such a condition. There are so few true nymphomaniacs—perhaps there are none—that the term has been dropped from the roster of psychosexual disorders. The candidate I saw was an exceptionally beautiful woman who required a different man every night. During the entire course of her adult life, over fifteen years, she had picked up a new one each evening that she was physically well enough to do so. She wanted no interference with her life-style from me. She couldn't change; she had no intention of trying. All she wanted to know was whether she had a dysfunction because she didn't have orgasms with everyone!

Perhaps there are more of these women than I know. The world of prostitution, massage parlors, sex clubs, and pornography must contain them, but the professionals who have consulted me generally want to know how to increase their sex drive, so that they can at least enjoy their work. A man employed at a sex club wants to know how he can have more frequent erections; a woman wants to know how she can stop feeling imposed on by the hands that reach and the bodies that intrude upon her. The closest to nymphomania that some women come may be to satisfy their exhibitionistic or dramatic needs by being photographed nude or during lovemaking. Still, this isn't the classic nymphomania we used to think existed, the woman who wanted sex all the time, cameras or not.

If nymphomania does not exist, hypersexuality does. There are times in people's lives when sex is likely to be the most common and sometimes the best defense against isolation or trouble. But hypersexual women suffering an identity crisis because of inadequate achievement, or failing at intimacy because of high achievement, have long since ceased to be perceived as nymphomaniacs. I've found that one questions their sexual health at one's own risk. To suggest to the "new" woman that she may be using sex to avoid other issues is to court her wrath, unless she herself realizes something is amiss and asks for help.

These people are to be distinguished from the sex addicts, those to whom sex is a "fix." Indeed, the narcotics analogy may have been proven apt when studies suggested that sexual relations may cause the body to release certain natural opiates—the recently discovered and much publicized antipain chemicals called enkephalins and endorphins. Thus sex, in addition to whatever else it does, may actually reduce pain and promote euphoria in much the same fashion as small doses of the morphinelike drugs. The sex addict, then, may literally be a junkie, in one sense.

The fantasy of the nymphomaniac will probably never die in the male consciousness. That wonderfully avid creature in pearls, garter belt, and high heels will continue to reflect the male desire for sexual indulgence without courtship. As a woman, I'm glad the fantasy can be played on from time to time. As a sex therapist, I'm relieved that real nymphomania doesn't seem to exist. It might be very difficult to treat.

On Homosexuality

TOGETHER WITH MOST of my sex therapist colleagues, I take cautious pride in saying, "I treat homosexuals who have sexual disorders just as I would treat any heterosexual. It makes no difference to me." Yet when my first homosexual patient, a young advertising executive, sat elegantly in my office some years ago, I wondered if I could do it. I did not question whether I could handle the intimate sexuality of two men; sexual acts are not that different between humans, no matter what the gender combination. My main concern was whether I could trust that my patient was truly homosexual merely because he said so. If I felt that he was really more heterosexual than homosexual, wasn't it my responsibility to help him back to "normality"? Should I do this before or after I helped him overcome his sexual disorder?

The problem resolved itself after I listened awhile to the young man. He was charming, capable, sexually troubled—and homosexual. There was no doubt. He enjoyed sex only with other men. He was so comfortable with his orientation that he set me at ease.

We didn't have guidelines for homosexual normality in those days. People who liked others of the same sex were considered psychiatrically deviant. The word *gay* had a flamboyant connotation, redolent of transvestite night life and other wanton states. Gay meant fey, girlish. Believing the serious, pleasant man in my chair to be normal was an act of faith, then.

As a beginning psychiatrist, I found drawing the line between homosexuality and heterosexuality as difficult as separating pornography from art, art from sham, sham from madness. Were there truly homosexual people, who didn't care sexually for members of the opposite sex yet could maintain orderly, even loving social relations with them? Were there any truly heterosexual people, who couldn't experience sexual attraction to human beings like themselves? What label should we affix to our own bodies and psyches, and could we trust the labels that others traveled under?

When this book was first written, the American Psychiatric Association had created a remarkable set of diagnostic criteria for evaluating homosexuality. By itself, they said, homosexuality was not a mental disorder. (This did not rule out the possibility of its being some form of physical or chemical abnormality.) It became a psychiatric disorder, however, said the APA, when homosexuals were persistently concerned about changing their orientation, when they had such strong negative feelings regarding homosexuality that they could neither enjoy it nor, in some cases, do more than fantasize about it.

Today, homosexuality as a diagnostic category is not mentioned in *DSM-IV*. It lurks only in the old index to *DSM-III-R*, where it was considered under Sexual Disorders Not Otherwise Specified. Example 3 was: persistent and marked distress about one's sexual orientation. Since this is no longer valid, one must conclude that homosexuality is not a psychiatric or sexual disorder and that people who are depressed or disturbed by their orientation suffer depression or anxiety, only.

It is really quite amazing that we still do not know any more about the causes of homosexuality than we used to know, say, about disease. Medicine once consisted largely of seeing and naming, observation and nomenclature. Profuse causes for illness were guessed at: the malodorous air, the muddy water, the phlegm and contagion of bad spirits. Later, when specific causal agents, like the tubercle bacillus, were identified, almost every visible disorder was attributed to them. Beriberi and lupus, for example, were thought to be forms of tuberculosis.

Not knowing what causes homosexuality, today we are still flailing about on the scientific floor and trying to find some leg of logic to stand on. We don't blame all emotional pain on the "latent homosexuality" virus any more because we now don't consider homosexuality an illness. Yet if it is not an illness, what is it?

We have studied the animal kingdom in order to prove that homosexual behavior exists there as a normal variant. "Animals do it all the time" used to be a favorite defense for homosexual behavior. "It must be natural."

Well, animals don't do that much of it. Creatures of the same sex do often mount one another, but the union is transitory. Such behavior increases when animals are crowded, or under stress, just as humans tend to hold on to one another for support when the pressure is high. Among people, contact at trying times probably becomes sexual more readily than it does among animals, who merely hang on to each other briefly in agitated confusion. In any event, students of animal behavior have told us that true homosexual mating, carried through to climax, is rare.

On the other hand, one wonders what these researchers mean

by "true homosexual mating." Are the brief encounters for which so many homosexuals cruise "true mating"? Or are they more like "mounting behavior"?

In June 1980, *Science* reported on female macaque monkeys mounting one another. Placed in a small cage, six female macaques first established the dominance of one of their number. This dominant macaque then had relations with a particular partner as though she were a male monkey. She even exhibited the male "ejaculation face," a round-mouthed expression, presumably of ecstasy.

Thus, under the stimulus of being crowded suddenly into a new environment, aggression and sexuality that terminated in coituslike behavior, with orgasm, emerged between females. The monkeys displayed a pattern of body contact under stress, mated according to dominance, and regularly experienced what appeared to be complete orgasm. Perhaps the predictable passions of animals can teach us something about the origins of homosexual behavior among men and among women who are crowded into large cities under stressful conditions. Still, we can't say for sure that stressful environment causes homosexuality. Perhaps it contributes.

Great names in analytic literature have written that the emotional conditions in a person's family abet homosexuality and perhaps cause it. They say that conflicts centered about dominance and submission remain too long the focus of the private life of the person in question. Their theories make good sense. Many homosexual relations—the sadist and masochist, the screamer and silencer, the servant and queen—seem like parodies of some earlier tension between parent and child. Yet many troubled homosexual relations are nothing like the dramas that such exhibitionists create. They are not caricatures. They are serious characterological struggles, as deeply embittering as those in any heterosexual union approaching desolation.

I don't think we can say that dominance-submission struggles in the nuclear family cause homosexuality. They cause damage. Sometimes they cause destruction. The route to becoming homosexual could not be so simple, else the world would be divided into two camps by now. Power struggles may contribute to the form homosexuality takes, but surely no one would credit them with being the singular cause.

Theorists about world power relations have spun intricate histories relating homosexuality to male-dominated or female-dominated societies through the millennia. Male-dominated societies are supposed to be rigid and authoritarian. Within them, homosexuality is feared and punished. Female-dominated societies, on the other hand, are said to tolerate it better. Perhaps today, one theorist ventures, we are moving toward a unisexual society, in which peace and pansexuality prevail because only the genitals are different.

Philosophers of world ecology suggest that homosexuality, as a natural method of population control, is sure to increase in response to the need. And a noted sociobiologist hints that the torch of the arts might not be passed from one generation to the next were it not for homosexual culturebearers. Nevertheless, history, ecology, family dynamics, and the animal kingdom have failed to provide either cause or absolution.

What have scientists been doing about this ignorance? Once again, as is customary in the first phase of any scientific effort, they have been observing and naming. While we all know that homosexuality is at least as old as ancient Greece, though rarely as respected as it was then, efforts to investigate it methodically have been extraordinarily few. Major projects in the past few decades have been directed at separating and making public the distinction between homosexuals, hermaphrodites, transsexuals, transvestites, and bisexuals.

The words *gender role* and *gender identity* have become very important in helping to distinguish people with diverse sexual patterns. Gender role, blurred today, involves what one does to indicate the degree to which one is male or female. Gender identity is the sense of knowing to which sex one belongs. Homosexual men usually have a male gender identity, though they may adopt "female" gender roles. They think of themselves as men, though some may perform what they perceive to be female acts.

Transsexuals think they have a gender identity opposite from that of the sex one would assign them on sight of their naked bodies.

The cross-dressers—transvestites—believe they are men, but love feminine garments, which arouse them. Women who dress in men's clothing are not usually called transvestites. For women, dressing in men's clothing is fashionable and not a sexual variation, no matter how sexy it makes the wearer feel.

Hermaphrodites, who have two sets of organs, will grow up believing they are whatever their parents call them. Bisexuals, mating with both sexes, usually consider themselves to be what they look like.

Some scientific work suggests that all this confusion begins in utero. Progestin-treated mothers have given birth to "tomboyish" girls, while mothers treated with the female hormone diethylstilbestrol have given birth to males with undescended testicles and fertility problems, as well as emotional difficulties. Some of these have preferred a homosexual orientation.

The drugs a mother takes during pregnancy may influence the sexual orientation of her child. So, perhaps, can anxiety and depression, which have druglike effects on the nervous system.

Studies in the '80s began to establish the supremacy of chemistry over nurture in the sexual test tube. The Division of Endocrinology at Cornell University Medical College then righted the world of confused identities by dosing eighteen male pseudohermaphrodites with androgen. These gentlemen had been raised unambiguously as girls. The male hormone caused seventeen to change to a male gender identity and sixteen to a male gender role. Still, we do not know what intrauterine factors—what alterations of chemistry within the womb—have made certain men through the centuries affect the same mincing gait and act out the same gross caricatures of the bitchy woman. We don't know why, chemically, other less outrageously styled people choose to attach themselves to same-sexed lovers. Most recently, it has been hypothesized that the size of the hypothalamus may be related to sexual orientation and geneticists are attempting to localize chromosomal sites, but without firm correlation.

To psychiatrists, it doesn't really matter that we do not know. Chemistry and world history are of no help when one directly confronts a patient. The question of what causes homosexuality recedes while one faces the troubled human being in the chair. We have little choice but to follow the lead of the early analysts by searching out the source of the anguish. Our goal is to relieve pain, not to change a person's sexual preference, although sometimes that may ensue.

After empathy, the question "Why?" becomes the strongest uncovering tool we have. Our first issue is not what causes this person's homosexuality, but rather what characterizes this human being's pain and why does he or she suffer it? The elegant young man is fast slipping into depression because he is not potent with his lover. His work and appetite are impaired; his lover has become abusive. But why should he want to become potent with a man whose response to impotence is aggression?

In another case, why does a young man who has just opened the homosexual closet for his parents' inspection insist on telling them the most shocking details of his subway sexuality? Why does he rouse them to fear and rage, so that his mother calls me every day to beg me to "change him back"?

Why does a famous lesbian patient want to give up her life because her lover has left her? Is she setting me up to want to desert her also?

Perhaps if we can negotiate the passions and find the reason, locate the crucial tender point, we will know what to do next.

The next step will not be concerned with changing homosexuality, but with understanding the drive to compulsive suffering, with asking why pain is so methodically embraced.

The pain may result from inevitable choices based on hating an opposite-sex parent while loving the same-sex parent. A nervous mother who abuses or overprotects her son may produce not only a homosexual male but a guilty one. He may wish to be punished for rejecting her. If his father is warmly affectionate, the stimulus to homosexuality is increased. The guilt of "stealing" father from mother adds to the need for punishment. And if the father cannot protect against the mother's invasiveness, women may seem an insurmountable enemy. Early experiences may teach people to expect the worst from half the human race forever.

In our time, no population has been more depleted by the lethal power of a virus. AIDS has cruelly devastated the homosexual community, which has contributed so much to culture, style and art. This has not altered my treatment approach. I help gay people feel less guilty about being loved, just like anyone else. I don't have to decide whether they are gay or not. The homosexual may suffer the very same emotional debacles that any ordinary, presbyopic, overweight, underdisciplined heterosexual may confront on the way to peace. At each step along the road, one decides for oneself which way to go.

The Matter of Smell

AS I WALK down the stairs to my office, I can sometimes smell my patients. One woman wears a rich, penetrating scent reminiscent of the thousand blossoms of empress trees in June. Whenever I detect it, I remember falling in love. Another wears a heavy gardenia perfume, almost edible. Gardenias were my parents' wedding flowers. I find myself momentarily wishing I was wearing white and getting married again. A third wears a preparation whose molecules are so arranged that they inspire me to want to don the high heels that I never wear except as a sexual indulgence. I haven't asked her the name of her mixture. It might be dangerous.

I wonder whether we, as male and female humans, have been trained by commerce to associate floral smells with romance and musky smells with aggressive, lusty sex. Or are we physiologically programmed to respond sexually to the gardens of spring, just as insects are drawn by odor and color to their petaled landing fields? Do we need nature to abet our sexual instincts because our creator neglected to complete our mating apparatus, or would we unite just as fervently without the May blossoms?

My hunch is that we all have an individual sexual scent. Certain other female organisms, after all, emit a mating substance that may be a very subtle odor attracting males. These chemicals are called "pheromones," and they are now used to control insect pest populations. The chemical is spread about at some distance from the crop. Males hurry to the spot, where they are put to death en masse. (Will human pheromones ever be used for a similar purpose?)

Some monkeys produce attractants called "copulins," specific for intercourse. Compounds like these may produce part of a woman's unique charm. Possibly copulins, in a mix of perspiration, bacteria, and skin oil, create a highly individual odor. Redheads are said to emit the sweetest and gentlest of such odors, brunettes the strongest, among white Americans.

Science has been at pains to extract or synthesize such a compound from humans. The researchers are really trying, encouraged by data suggesting that men respond to female sexual invitation far more often than women respond to male sexual pressure—it could be pheromones. Scientists prepared a love potion consisting of the suspected acids-of-attraction found in vaginal secretions. Women applied these to their chests at night so that men might sniff their way to more passion. Nothing special happened. The authors of the article about this experiment, in a burst of levity unusual for scientists, advised readers not to hold their breath in fear of pheromones.

For some time, researchers have titillated us with assertions that one substance or another in human sweat promotes menstrual regularity or synchrony, assists positive mood (ER-670 and ER-830), or enhances sexual attractiveness (dihydroepiandrosterone). To my knowledge, none of the substances has been shown to exert any directly observable sexually stimulating effect on human genitalia or consciousness.

The perfume industry has adapted such chemicals to be applied above the upper lip as love potions close to the vomeronasal organ (VNO), the pheromone receptor present in many mammals and possibly functional in the human upper respiratory tract as well. At this time, the main attractive effect of these chemicals may be to a customer's cash, as it is drawn out of pocket and into the purchase of expensive elixirs.

What about the odors we actually can smell? If researching the invisible attractant has failed so far, what can we say about those odors available to our noses?

Most human odor is caused by the action of bacteria. Not by accident. Our sweat and secretory glands, in company with the hair that surrounds them, are considered to be "scent organs"; they are found only in man, not in other mammals. Historically, humankind has sought to disguise those odors where it could not destroy them, although it is said that Napoleon would inform Josephine of his arrival a few days in advance so that she might be warned not to wash. Some men take to the perfume of blood, sweat, and urine the way connoisseurs enjoy strong cheeses and aged meat. Smells are said to be an important part of the earthy life, though I would guess that there are more women unaware of their aroma and more men afraid to say they are put off by a strong scent than otherwise.

Traveling to the opposite end of the cleanliness scale, we find men who wash before sex, wash after sex, and some who even wash during. One patient whom I treated kept a crock of water at his bedside to bathe his genitals—his wife's hands sometimes had cooking odors on them. Of course, he also bathed immediately after oral sex or intercourse. There are no statistics, but I sense that the cleanliness fetish is becoming as common among men as it is among women. More men in our generation may be repelled by female odor than in the past. We have come some distance from those times when cleanliness was considered so sissified that doctors refused to rinse their hands before plunging them into women's vaginas, thus killing many in "childbed fever."

The controversy over whether or not our "natural" odors are sexual attractants or repellants continued at the time this book was written with almost as much vigor as the dispute over whether or not females were interested in sex at all times. We still have no answer. Proponents of the positive view allowed little argument. Dr. C. Owen Lovejoy wrote on "The Origin of Man" in *Science* that human females were "continually sexually receptive." He expressed no doubt. He was almost as certain that the "redolent individuality" of underarm and urogenital scents assisted mating and pair-bonding through an assertion of sexual uniqueness. As an anthropologist, Dr. Lovejoy may be correct. As a sex therapist, I find human beings often to be very much out of touch with what may—or may not—be their sexual nature.

Perhaps our nasal sensitivity is fast becoming extinct. Perhaps we are something like those laboratory hamsters who show defects in mounting and ejaculation when the nerves to their olfactory apparatus are destroyed. We smoke, drink, and live in polluted cities where sinusitis and other nasal complaints are endemic. By adulthood, most tobacco-smoking urbanites are so nasally stunted that only the strongest odor of bacterial decay or the heaviest dose of perfume will reach them.

More optimistically, if the olfactory sense of our race is dying out, it may be because we hardly need it for self-protection or for love. For even without copulins or pheromones or any musky substances that males may produce to string us along, there is no shortage of sexual communication. After speech, posture, and clothing—and maybe electrical current and heat waves—I would bank on the eyes to carry the message.

Overeating and Sex

I DID NOT begin to treat people for their obesity by design. Specializing in sex was enough. I had no ambition to explain calorie countdowns and exercise equivalents to individuals who could very well understand those simplicities for themselves. Yet I am becoming as intrigued by the pleasures and pathologies of eating as I am by the diversities of lovemaking. They are very much alike.

Right now I have four overweight women in my practice. Two are obese; one used to be immense; the fourth has a borderline weight problem. They were referred to me for treatment mainly for their sexual difficulties and only incidentally for their over-weight. Two of them feel that if they could ever lose weight, their thin, sexual selves would emerge. That might be a disaster, because they wouldn't know how to handle either sexual attention or their own impulses. The other two worry mainly because they feel no sexuality, no urgency beneath the upholstery. They pay me to help them to experience libido, to encourage them to quest for romance, to want to have intercourse. Meanwhile, they are fat because, since sex isn't in prospect at the moment, being attractive doesn't matter.

For me, understanding the complex connection between sexual difficulty and fat is a fascinating challenge.

Many thinkers have related obesity and sexuality. The first psychoanalysts, especially the Freudians, had a great concern about the things that went into and came out of the human body early in life and later. They had the idea that we could mix up the functions of our orifices and gain pleasure at one end of the body from what ought to be giving us pleasure at the other. Since then several psychiatrists, like Hilde Bruch, have thought deeply about the sexual implications of eating too much. Yet few general physicians include a focus on their patients' sexual functions or psychology as part of their treatment of obesity. They prescribe diets and diet pills. They recommend "behavior mod." Very few authorities have attempted to formulate treatment plans that deal with the sexual psychology of obesity. Perhaps the subject of fat is so intimately related to sex that we are embarrassed by it. Thus our sexual hang-ups, continuing in spite of the sexual revolution, may be killing us.

Obesity is a national health problem of major proportions. When people weigh more than 20 percent over normal, their health is at risk. Up to 30 percent of men and 40 percent of women are taking this risk. Almost one third of our population, 70 million people, could significantly improve their health by dieting! Disorders that are either aggravated or caused directly by obesity include osteoarthritis, especially of the hips, and sciatica. Fat people also suffer more diabetes, varicose veins, thromboembolisms, ventral and hiatal hernias, gallstones, and hypertension than do people of normal weight. They are seriously courting coronary artery disease and stroke. The dangers of being fat rival those caused by cancer. Certainly there is a powerful negative dynamic at work here.

It is popular to say that people overeat to suppress sexual urges, but that may be an underestimation. I suspect that the majority of eating disorders result from sexual disorders. There is, however, a medical faction that argues the opposite—that problems with obesity cause sexual problems. Surgeons, especially, like this viewpoint. In a recent study called "Massive Obesity and Sexual Activity," thirteen men and ten women who were to undergo surgery that would partially prevent digestion— so that they could lose weight—were found to be sexually normal but ashamed of their obesity, which made them self-conscious. Perhaps so. On the other hand, many such patients find ways to fatten up again after surgery, some by drinking milkshakes all day. We ought to be able to distinguish a genetic need to be fat from a compulsion to eat to avoid sex. We ought to be able to predict better whether such drastic surgery will work. I have serious reservations about treating obesity as a physical disease that can be surgically corrected by removing a significant portion of a person's digestive system.

Eating and sexuality are related in at least three important ways: feelings related to the act of consumption, feelings associated with the sense of fullness, and those disturbed emotions accompanying the obesity itself.

The most prevalent disorder, the act of excessive eating, of continually placing food in one's mouth, tasting, chewing, and swallowing, so resembles intercourse that the most successful sex manual of the last decade took its title from a cookbook. A sexually troubled woman may easily make the transition from being afraid to fill her vagina to cramming her mouth with alternative delights. Men may confuse lust with rapacious appetite (a common cliché) or sublimate their longings for a vagina of their own by excessively appreciating the intake of food. Both men and women may use the act of eating to distract from sexual urges; sexual hunger may become permanently confused with a call to the larder. As odd as these mix-ups may sound to laymen, they do not surprise psychiatrists. We human beings possess so many brain circuits that it's a wonder more of them don't get crossed.

The act of eating, then, consists of desire with salivation, the excitement of tasting and chewing, and the orgasmic contractions of swallowing, repeated again and again. No physical act we perform is so like sexual union. People eat compulsively to excess in order to distract themselves pleasurably from pain. While busy chewing and eating and thinking about food, they have little room in their psyches for sexual longings, for fears of intimacy, self-assertion, and dependence, or for anger and grief. They swallow and reach, swallow and reach. Their blood goes to the stomach instead of perfusing the brain, as it might have were they trying to solve their problems. They think of food first on awakening and last before going to sleep at night.

Jane Brody, in the *New York Times*, wrote early about a disease she felt was sweeping the country: bulimarexia. This means alternately stuffing (bulimia) and starving (anorexia). Much like binge drinking, or drug addiction with periodic detoxification, this disease exacts a large price from body chemistry and hormonal balance. Some theorizers about anorexia nervosa suggest that a need to control (and stop) the body's growth and development is a cause of that disease. My own experience with approximately ten anorectics revealed conflict about emergent sexuality to be a core issue. Only when they had begun to allow themselves to feel sexual were they able to eat properly. This, however, involved dealing with all kinds of secondary issues, too.

Psychoanalysts dwell on still another type of gratification: sucking at mother's breast. If we enjoyed it, they say, we may always wish to return. It interests me that the men in my practice who had feeding conflicts with their mothers—for example, who were forced to eat when they were not particularly hungry—often have difficulty with sexual intimacy later. For them, to suckle a woman's breast means to give in to her dominance, to be a baby. It's a curious world.

The second part of the eating sequence, the fullness phase, also has obvious sexual implications. Feeling surfeited may resemble having had an orgasm. It may also resemble having a large penis inside, or feeling pregnant. Distention effectively reduces the desire for intercourse. Certainly nausea, flatulence, constipation, diarrhea, and all the consequences of overeating reduce sexual eagerness. At the same time they activate or distend the digestive system, which is located near the sexual organs. Many obese people are overconcerned with their digestion. Their frequent bowel movements and urinations are probably erotically pleasurable. Anorectic patients too may derive sexual stimulation from their digestive systems. A colleague of mine was frequently called on to disimpact a young anorectic patient. This meant loosening and breaking up the hard bolus of stool inside her rectum. Later, when the patient and I analyzed it, she realized that when she disimpacted herself, it was a form of masturbation. When my colleague did it for her, it was sexually gratifying.

The fullness phase of eating may also be disordered because of an inability to experience it. Many fat people can't tell when they are stuffed with food. Just as they may be anesthetized to their sexual sensations, so they may not receive their abdominal messages. They shut out this area of their body as a source of pleasure and sensation, both sexually and digestively. Their "set point" is not functioning.

People rarely set out to get fat. They gain weight more by indirection. If they are too fat to be alluring, all the torments of attempt and rejection may be avoided. So may the dangers of intimacy. If one never gets close enough to others to express angry feelings, these, too, can be suppressed. Fat keeps people away from one another both literally and figuratively.

The elder analysts have elaborated under what difficulty people learn to eat, drink, and go to the toilet. The famous old Teutonic governesses destroyed their charges' later love lives by instilling habits of overcontrol; the all-allowing mothers of two decades ago had children who have had trouble maintaining stability in their sexual and economic lives, or so the theory goes. By extension of this kind of thinking, the man whose mother thought of him as an undernourished starveling may spend his adult life overeating to please her. The woman whose grandfather fed her sweets and kisses may seek metaphorically to return to those marzipan days for the rest of her adult life. Or the daughter whose father praised her cooking and joined her in feasting may turn her married domesticity into a vast orgiastic groaning board.

The variations are endless, but all lead to the same high reading on the scales. That which pleased us most profoundly in our childhood, or those ways in which we sought approval then, remain to protect us from desolation as long as we live. For these memories of happiness, we may risk our lives. It has been said that 80 percent of all efforts at dieting fail. The invisible opponent is love.

On Masturbation

I HAVE BEEN searching for a word to replace *masturbation* ever since starting to study the practice. All the synonyms—*self-stimulation, self-gratification, self-satisfaction*—sound awkward and mechanical. *Self-pleasuring* has come and gone, I think. Even though *to pleasure* is a perfectly acceptable verb, it seems like a euphemism. For some obscure linguistic reason, the Latin past participle *masturbatum* was never reduced to "masturb," the way *perturbatum* and *disturbatum* were shortened to produce "perturb" and "disturb." Perhaps people hadn't talked about autoeroticism enough to need the short form until recently.

As we know, our Victorian ancestors created the notion of "the solitary vice," which was not only a form of "self-abuse" but constituted a threat to society. Masturbation was considered a demoralizing waste of vitality and semen, causing insanity, destroying the matrimonial sentiment, and mutilating desire. It blighted the growth of sex organs and resulted in deformity and ugliness. Vulgarity, sickness, sorrow, and shame were the inevitable consequences of this terrible and addicting habit.

169

Today, while there are a few who believe that the solitary vice should be a public virtue—who say that it creates sanity and high morale, satisfies desire, encourages the development of sex organs, and results in happiness and inner and outer beauty—most of us, or most of my patients, at least, want to know what part it really ought to play in life, and more particularly, how it relates to the treatment of their disorder. They have read the family books on sex and know that masturbation is healthy if it's not a sole sexual outlet. They tell their children that it's all right as long as it's private. But what about them? Will it help or hinder their quest for sexual improvement?

In good psychiatric tradition, one answers questions with questions. I ask my patients: "When did you begin to masturbate? How, specifically, do you do it? Do you have orgasms? When do you find yourself masturbating most? When is masturbation least on your mind? Why do you think that is? Do you enjoy masturbating? What role do you think it plays in your mental and physical health and your appreciation of sex?"

The answers to these questions form a pattern depending on the disorder. My nonorgasmic women patients rarely masturbate, or if they do gently pleasure themselves, they tend to have started late in life. Women able to have orgasms, but not during intercourse, are usually reasonably adept at it. Women who have orgasms during intercourse with some men but not with others (without understanding why) frequently have limited masturbatory experience. Those who suffer vaginismus often masturbate to orgasm easily.

As for men, premature ejaculators tend to masturbate not for joy but for release of tension. Retarded ejaculators often masturbate compulsively, addicted to a too-frequent habit. Impotent men fall into no category that bears generalization. The psychology of impotence is too diverse.

As a sex therapist, I may teach the inexperienced how to

masturbate. I may encourage practiced people to share their solitary experiences, to learn to masturbate in the company of their partners. For a woman, masturbation during intercourse is often a large step toward coital satisfaction.

I also teach those women who tighten their vaginal muscles too firmly to admit a penis that they can voluntarily loosen their vagina enough to allow entry; this is accomplished with masturbationlike techniques.

Premature ejaculators may be taught to delay their ejaculations on masturbation as on intercourse. Retarded ejaculators usually need to learn to reduce their masturbatory frequency, especially those who do so in the twenty-four to forty-eight hours before intercourse. They also often need to learn to give up being so much in control of themselves and others, sometimes by becoming premature ejaculators for a while. And while impotent men do not, in my experience, have a "most frequent" masturbatory pattern, they may occasionally alleviate their impotence by using masturbation fantasies during relations with their partners.

But what is masturbation, and what does one expect people to do when one instructs them to masturbate? Scholarship in the field is limited. There are no histories, no significant bodies of literature. My sociobiology textbook doesn't include it in the index, perhaps because most animals do not have hands that can reach their genitals. Anthropologists observe it from time to time. Some statistics exist about what percentage of ordinary people do it, but what precisely do they do? Perhaps Philip Roth wrote about it best, making the point in *Portnoy's Complaint* that they do just about everything.

Educational films exist showing what acts different people perform. They demonstrate that masturbatory behavior is much like that in everyday life. A thespian stimulates himself with dramatic gestures, uttering cries as he reaches crescendos of not quite believable ecstasy; a plump female uses a variety of vibrators with the button-pushing skills she might have acquired on a dishwasher or a microwave oven. In a scientific film, a woman reads an erotic book while methodically stimulating her clitoris with her index and middle fingers, thus producing an orgasm. The film also shows graphs of her blood pressure, pulse rate, and other parameters of excitement and climax. Pornographic films usually demonstrate a nameless man's firm grip on his member, his hand moving back and forth at varying speeds until the ejaculatory spurt. Women in most of the pornography that I have seen masturbate with the same efficiency displayed by the erotic female specimen in the scientific film. Detachment is crucial. Another kind of detachment is offered by those proselytizers for masturbation who attempt a clean, inspirational approach through relaxation and meditation.

My patients are different. They are neither detached, efficient, nor inspired. Inexperienced women mostly grope in the dark toward some flash of good feeling that they do not know how to sustain. Often they do not even feel comfortable using their hands, but find instead some favorite or convenient object like a teddy bear, a book, or a pillow, against which they move with irregular passion. Sometimes they have orgasm. More often they don't. And there are actually men and women who have never touched their genitals because their religion or upbringing forbids them to. One man I treated had not ejaculated in all the twenty-eight years of his life, though once he began, he functioned normally.

Masturbation, then, is anything we do to excite ourselves sexually, toward orgasm, without help from anyone else. Depending on character, we may be timid, methodical, inventive, or daring in our choice of stimuli. Depending on personal history, what excites us may be oral, genital, anal, or general. It's our own game. And when I help people to learn masturbation,

I cannot tell them to press this and jiggle that in some prescribed sequence. Once they have a good understanding of their anatomy, we try to go on to devise an emotional and physical sequence that is suited to their needs and nature.

Ultimately, the question is, Why do people masturbate? Until we know why to do it, trying to learn how seems foolish. Children may stimulate themselves simply because it feels good. That is reason enough for adults also, but if they are not free to feel good genitally, one may be required to approach the problem's complexities rather than its simplicities.

People who do not masturbate are frequently unable not only to touch themselves but also to enjoy life's other satisfactions. For them, pleasure is often understood as sin. They are the audience to whom much of the recent sexual literature is addressed. They are also the people least able to profit by purely sexual instruction. Most need help first in simply feeling pleasure without guilt—in buying attractive clothes, delighting in nature, sleeping late, listening to music, even eating for the fun of it. All of a therapist's wariness and stoicism may be required to help a person experience forbidden happiness and translate that feeling into sexual arousal. The scales of guilt, self-denial, martyrdom, shame, and humiliation must be removed, one by one, each loss causing the sufferer a new pain, a new vulnerability. The price of pleasure is occasionally very high for both of us, as patients rage at not receiving love in the aberrant or truncated forms to which they are accustomed.

I do not usually try to teach the complex uses of masturbation. Patients tend to pick them up by themselves, once they have got the idea. They discover masturbation when they are lonely, tired, or bored. They may try it to relieve tension or stress or anger. Not uncommonly, masturbation finds a role in the salving of loss or in the process of mourning. Most of us recognize its usefulness as a source of comfort before sleep at night.

Masturbation also tends to serve a special function in freeing fantasy. People who do not allow themselves mental journeys during intercourse may travel wherever it is they want to go during self-stimulation. If loving someone else excludes lewdness, then lewdness may be the mainstay of masturbatory fantasy, or vice versa. People may indulge their homosexual thoughts, too, or their concerns with urine and feces when by themselves, as they might not do with others. The masturbatory event may become a truly private world, not intended to be shared. Masturbation also frequently serves amour. It may accompany the anticipation of a forthcoming encounter or assist the fond recollection of a good time past. It may reduce the frustration of not possessing someone we desire by allowing us to make love in fantasy, if not reality.

The first aim of masturbation is an affirmation of self-love, of assurance to ourselves that we are worthy of joy even if no one else gives it to us or even if we choose not to accept the sexual love that someone proffers. As such, the freedom to masturbate is part of our liberation. We are entitled to do what we want, for ourselves. Whether we share our sexuality becomes a matter of choice, not obligation. Most men take this freedom for granted, but many women need to be taught. It is part of the code of values that a sex therapist imparts. Our most private freedoms reflect the temper of our age, the history that shapes us, the events that we shape.

Yet for most of us, the ultimate message of masturbation is still a longing for someone else. We are not ready to go it alone, no matter how convincingly the ecologists or the acolytes of celibacy speak. We may masturbate in early life, and we may be required to pleasure ourselves at the feeble end of it, but most of the time we tend to prefer making love.

Sex as Recreation

I GREW UP, summers, as a hotel brat. My mother owned a resort, a white stucco vacation palace in the Catskill Mountains. It was there I learned that sex was recreation. Only much later in life did I realize that sex might involve complicated feelings.

Sex was what everyone did in the afternoon when they went to "rest." They did it late at night, too. I could tell by the sounds coming out of windows and through paneled doors to hallways. There were two hundred rooms. Sometimes the couples left their doors open to get a breeze. Everyone did it with everyone else. Married women did it with busboys and waiters while their husbands were working in the city. Everyone knew. Day camp counselors did it with one another, mostly, like parents. The musicians did it with the most attractive women guests, and the master of ceremonies was king of the harem. After him came the lifeguard. Everyone knew that, too.

I had a very simple sort of childhood.

Sex was fun.

Or so it seemed. The realities may have become obscured by the patina of time, but even though I didn't leave the hotel until I was well into adulthood, I don't remember arguments about sex, or deep, psychic troubles about performance, or any particular struggles to preserve virginity or avoid infidelity.

What I often find myself doing as a psychiatrist and sex therapist is teaching people that sex can be play. While I have learned quite a bit about the serious aspects of lust, procreation, jealousy, malfunction, and all of that, I find myself laughing at memories of the Rabelaisian scenes of my childhood and trying to convey that in sex as in other realms of life profound purpose is not always absolutely essential, and that delight, relaxation, and sensual pleasure are perfectly adequate goals in themselves.

People come to me and ask how they can make their sex lives more fun. I can't suggest that they go to the Catskills, which are very ethnic and hardly exist as a recreation center any longer. (My mother, who recently celebrated sixty-five years of running her resort—she is nearly ninety years old—reports that the guests are as lively, but not as conspicuously lusty, as they used to be.) I couldn't prescribe swinging even in the '70s—it could be chancy psychologically, even perilous—though I didn't necessarily proscribe it. Today, in the era of AIDS, I would forbid it if I could. Even in the heyday of sexual freedom, I never noticed people having much fun at the sex clubs. Mostly they took drugs and went about their sexual Olympics with forced good spirits. And today, unless people think of it themselves, I don't recommend pornography. Ways to have sexual "fun" are up to individuals, as consenting adults, to select for themselves. I can only mention that they exist.

When I treat a joyless couple, I may ask if they crave romance, love, lust, or adventure. In one case, the man wanted gentle loving; the woman could barely control an appetite for lust and adventure. (Most of the time it is the other way around.) It turned out that the man was suffering severe anxiety attacks—he was concerned about his job and other nonsexual matters. His heart palpitated and his palms went cold with sweat at night. He wanted sex as comfort. His anxiety, however, made his wife furious, and she was ready to discharge her rage in lusty adventure with other men. When I worked with the sources of his anxiety and taught her to soothe him, to help him relax before starting relations, their sex life resumed as a pleasantly satisfactory, if not entirely aphrodisiac, experience. When the anger at his helplessness subsided and she found that she could calm him, she was willing, even eager, to settle for pleasant sex and containable dreams of romance. The first route to "fun," then, is understanding the problem that destroys it. That accounts for most of my therapeutic work.

In addition to psychotherapy, I often give one piece of practical advice. It is the lesson I learned during all those summer vacations. I preach that planning is a cardinal principle of good sex. My patients object, saying that recreational sex ought to be "spontaneous." Personally, I think the search after sexual "spontaneity"—especially in households thronging with children, in-laws, delivery boys, repairmen, and strangers asking directions—is a lost cause. But even if there are only two at home, married couples, like lovers in the most intense phase of infatuation, might profit by planning their affairs.

The practice of dating can continue throughout life. I suggest that people should arrange their amatory meetings. If they put aside what is bothering them—exams, difficult teachers, taxes, mortgages, other partners—they might even have a good time. People whose partners won't do this with them often go off and find someone else to do it with. Trysting, after all, is a form of dating. The outcome is generally sexual, and the event is extramarital—or at least extracurricular—for at least one partner. Anticipation plays a large role in its excitement. Preparation also contributes to a sense of fulfillment. Nothing could be less spontaneous. In this highly scheduled era, couples need to set time and place. Serendipitous haystacks and moments in the barn loft under the swallow's nest don't pop up anymore for most of us.

As far as I have been able to determine, the most common ingredients of a tryst are some sort of a bed, some mild chemical relaxant like wine, perhaps music, and about three hours of free time. This formula for optimal sex transcends economic and social classifications. If one had a bird's-eye view of a city, with all apartments and hotel rooms visible, those having sex this way would far outnumber any other. Yet, as simple as this formula is, many people who come to a sex therapist in order to recapture sexual bliss, or at least the feeling of having fun together, have forgotten it. They postpone their sex to the last failing moments of the day. They try to be "spontaneous" after the ten o'clock news, while visions of televised disaster and mayhem still dance in their heads and the grease on the dinner dishes has long since hardened like candle wax. They are tired. What they need is a long bath, a heavy sleep, and a few erotic dreams. They aren't up to anything else.

I encourage married couples to take time off and meet each other on workday afternoons, the way they would if they were having an affair. I suggest long weekends away—not in the country house (if there is one), where repairing and meal-making are required—but at an inn or a friend's home. Diversity and planning help to make life more of a party.

Beyond establishing time and place, there are also a variety of other incidental ways in which sex can consciously be made more fun. Dancing can be part of foreplay, or even of the act, itself. Being in good condition helps, too, although not all of us can aspire to athletic sexual variations. The setting, while basically often the same, can be varied, according to one's mood, with candles, flowers, firelight (if possible), perfume, incense, plants, pillows, or any other atmospheric device. Some people prefer mirrored disco balls and flashing neon for effect; others like a clear view of moon, stars, and blinking planes through a skylight. Contrary to some opinion, the greater the variety of senses involved in a sexual encounter, the more pleasure. Sight, sound, and touch all enhance sensation.

Perhaps more important than any blueprint for pleasure is a person's mood. I think most of us require a change of pace after a day's not so frolicsome striving. The exchange of anxieties that passes for intimacy among many couples is really another and subtler form of doing battle, and is hardly arousing. One lesson I teach is that people can, under most circumstances, control their moods.

Couples often seem to marry because they laugh and have fun together. Then they promptly forget how to do it. Yet there are so many ways. They all involve a deliberate and emotionally mature effort to set aside trouble. One can laugh at another's jokes, mimicries, or skewed viewpoint of the nature of life. People can create comic dialogues or rejoice in plain being silly. What starts as horsing around can end as intense affection or the deepest coital love. Although Dr. Johnson said that a man cannot spend his life in frolic, Horace reminded us that it is pleasant to act foolishly in the right place. When Kissinger said that power is the ultimate aphrodisiac, he spoke for the solemn and grim-faced mask of passion. The other face of the mask, the comic perspective, may be a more universally seductive prescription—and certainly more fun.

On Incest

THE THOUGHT OF incest rouses an odd mixture of repugnance and curiosity in many of us. As I consider this response, I remember how the sexual revolution changed people's views of incest, and how that affected my role as a therapist. Incest did not become a cause until recently. The newspapers are now filled with controversy over recovered memories. Movies with incestuous themes have begun to appear. Pornography openly exploits it. Novels deal directly with it now, rather than as a fantasy or unconscious motivation. And the world of domestic justice, social work, foster homes—all that vast caretaking machinery coping with our tragedies—is inundated with the problem. It fills their official publications and takes up the hours in their casebooks. Incest has not become a way of life or a political issue. It is a national dilemma. I work best with individual complexities, the acts we perform without knowing precisely what we are doing. I struggle with our tendency to flay ourselves for what we assume are our sins. Early in my career, I had to decide upon my attitude toward incest. I suspect it is the same view that I hold today.

I was called upon to treat the case of a man suffering depression after the end of a fifteen-year relationship with his daughter. He had first made love to her when he was thirty-two and she was twelve. How could he have done it? He deserved to be depressed. Why should I relieve him of his just retribution?

Yet when I met the grieving, loving man who wanted his daughter to be happy with her new husband, who did not want to impose his misery on her, I remained silent and listened. I tried to let myself get in touch with the depths of feeling that may bind all fathers and daughters at levels beyond convention, whether or not they ever sound those bottom waters. Our incestuous feelings are, perhaps, the essence of that organism we call the family; they are the union we cannot act out with our bodies, the romance we may not fulfill.

This father was genuinely mourning the loss of a person he loved. Though that love was expressed sexually, he had also given his daughter the rest of his life—his nurture, his loyalty, his possessions. Had he been an old Egyptian pharaoh, an Inca ruler, or a native of certain Pacific islands, his union would have been blessed. He would not have had to experience this grief. I tried to remember these things as I worked with his guilt and loneliness.

Students of the family tell us that incest mainly occurs in two types of families, the antisocial and the rigidly conforming. The former, the "acting-out" families, seem the natural breeders of disaster. Incest goes with truancy, thievery, addiction, neglect, and assault. We easily attribute the behavior to the disorganization and maladjustment of such a family, separated from societal norms. When court decisions must be made as to what to do with offending parents, simple solutions like separating them from their children are generally resorted to.

But what about the private, law-abiding families? Incestuous bonds are different in these. In such family groups, incest does not usually occur because of random lust. An arrangement of physical and emotional circumstances often leads to its inevitability. In the example of the fifteen-year bond mentioned earlier, the mother was a bedded invalid; the father saw it as his duty to be home. Their mutual care of mother and the household led to a "marriage" between father and child that was terminated only when the daughter resolved to leave her father and start a family of her own.

In another family that I treated, where the father was domineering and cruel, a sister and brother were driven to unite by a need to express their undercurrent rage and to have each other's love. What should be decided when cases like these surface because of a neighbor's observation or a child's sudden awareness of wrongdoing? The answers are not simple.

Within such families, brother-sister incest is most common, according to Gebhart and Kinsey. Father-and-daughter coupling occurs with the next greatest frequency. Unions between mothers and sons are immensely rare; fathers and sons, and mothers and daughters, are the rarest. Other pairings—uncles and nieces, fathers and stepchildren, have not been extensively quantified.

Even without statistics, one would guess that brother-sister incest was most frequent because of their proximity and availability to one another. Between siblings, one must distinguish between incest as sexual exploration and as an established relationship. Exploration between siblings is usually an extension of natural curiosity. Yet many people come to psychiatrists (or go to their graves) with an extraordinary burden of guilt for a few childhood escapades that were more educational than sexual. The same is true of "incestuous" homosexual relations. Events that only occur a few times, or for short periods, and that do not interfere with further efforts at making love outside the family, seem within the bounds and part of the process of growing up. On the other hand, not even truly deviant and repetitive incestuousness behavior can be treated summarily as a punishable offense, a situation in which the guilty pair must be separated immediately. Abrupt action can cause more damage than the offense it seeks to remedy.

Some people include forced sexual relations and those accompanied by violence under the heading of incest. I believe that a distinction between rape and incest needs to be made in these cases. Incestuous rape and incest accompanied by violence differ from the gentler seductions that create the more subtle predicaments. Incestuous violence should be considered as a kind of rape, I think, because the sexual act is motivated more by brutality than by family attraction. I have the conviction that violence not exerted in self-defense is always a crime and that victims ought to be separated from their violators as the lesser of two evils, no matter what the psychological dependence may have become. A daughter who must survive in a family where she is regularly beaten and sexually abused by a parent or sibling is better off away from all that. Even though we do not have the means to enforce justice or provide psychiatric care, I do not think we should let our consciences idle as society allows this destructiveness to go on. And we do allow it to go on. Studies indicate there are about 360,000 cases of childhood sexual abuse a year, roughly 38 percent of them incest. Among these cases, we do not know the incidence of forced or violent incest, but it must be extremely high; otherwise the acts would not have made the grade of becoming a statistic. Quiet, hidden incest probably does not get reported very often.

Sex therapists deal mainly with the problems of peaceful incest brought to them by the conforming families. For example, a beautiful young girl, who grew up essentially unsupervised among five brothers on a large Connecticut estate, was the willing recipient of her brothers' sexual energies from the age of ten to fourteen. When she realized her brothers' odd behavior, she became morbidly reclusive. She was brought to me by her busy, negligent mother, who told me that "the poor thing needs some cheering up and bringing out." She needed quite a lot more than that.

Children get involved in incest because it's urged on them and they do not know that it is not acceptable. They also learn to use sexuality with adults who will not respond to other approaches. They employ sexual strategies to gain affection from a parent or to disarm a rival sibling. When I was consultant to the New York Association for the Blind, a social worker told me that babies were born who learned to cry without tears because their blind parents could not see them, and other babies were born who learned to cry without screaming because their deaf parents could not hear them. If infants can be that perceptive, children can be terrifyingly accurate in selecting that behavior designed to produce response. Sex can win, in the family as in life, where achievement, character, purpose, and persistence all fail.

Sometimes parents perform sex acts with their children as the lone method of expressing affection. Their psyches have been so damaged that they can feel affection only as sex. Arousal creates their sole path for relating warmly to children or anyone else.

Sex can be power, dependence, or submission between relatives as between friends. A man may seduce his daughter out of hostility to his wife, who provides neither freedom nor sexual outlet. He can do it without leaving home or causing suspicion, for usually he can intimidate his child sufficiently not to reveal their secret. A mother may train her sons to erotic responses by masturbating them from the time they nurse at her breast, in the hope that they will grow up and never leave her to loneliness.

Incestuous sex can also be immensely loving, as when an adult brother and sister decide that they must live together, without the world knowing that they are lovers. I have also seen siblings who deny themselves incestuous love, even though they are so obviously suited for one another and so attracted that they cannot feel sexual toward others. Instead they care for one another with a devotion that borders the saintly.

Much has been written about the damage done by incest. Some studies, however, have individualized the experience more. Researchers have said that the repercussions of early incestuous experience may not cause obvious symptomatology until later in life (if, one must add, at all). The effects of a gentle exchange between an incestuous pair may, indeed, cause more anguish to the elder initiator than to the younger lover. The older person often feels the stigma of guilt and shame more intensely than the young person who participated with less awareness. Often the elder has the guilt, too, of not discouraging a child's attempts at incest.

Sometimes incest can be a stopgap even though other routes to love would be more socially and psychologically acceptable. A daughter devoted to the care of her sick parents from the time she was sixteen years old made love to a visiting uncle until both parents died. Then she felt free to go out into the world to make her own choice of lovers. Her uncle had sustained her emotionally and physically. He made it possible for her to live without deserting or upsetting her parents. He helped her to take a lifelong pleasure in lovemaking. She consulted me because she wanted to know if this experience might have an adverse effect on her own forthcoming marriage—if her past was fair to her future husband! Even the naïve participant in incest may suffer a huge burden of guilt.

Of course, when incest is combined with violence, the result may be a lifelong fear of sex and an inability to experience sexual tenderness. Violence to a child damages most because it may leave the victim forever unable to experience the most civilized emotions of mankind. More than fear of violence, it may instill a fear of love, which is the ultimate human degradation.

If I attempt to relieve the guilt of incestuous people, it does not necessarily mean that I approve of incest or decry the taboo. Incest taboos would appear to be a permanent condition of life, like birthing and dying. They are good for the survival of the race. In treating incest, the role of the psychiatrist is inevitably that of the physician—to reserve judgment and heal wounds.

Interlude: Laughter, Tears, and Orgasm

ONE IMPRESSION I get from the forty hours a week I spend with my patients, week after week, is that the most neglected sexual art these days is laughter—true mirth. Orgasm has become a very serious business. Men watch and count their partners' peaks and have begun to tabulate their own. Women throw their heads back, try hard, and agonize to reach yet another climax. Few seem aware of the aphrodisia of laughter—that laughing, fully and to the point of tears, can encourage and even prolong pleasure.

When my patients speak of orgasm, they tend to echo current manuals. They dwell on quantity rather than quality, success rather than meaning, sensation rather than emotion. If the ancients attempted to explain the human condition through epic narratives, the moderns seem preoccupied with brief definitions. They demand the bottom line.

But numbers fail to comprehend the subtleties of climax. As for the philosophy of orgasmic achievement, it feels good to get there quickly and easily, but what then, and so what? Nor does high sensation suffice as the aim of orgasm. The cult of hedonism is a frail substitute for the tradition of humanism. Over two decades of sexologists have promoted a creed—simplistic and redundant: "Success in the pleasure of sex requires that you allow yourself to enjoy." Such gurus knew about breathing and stroking and the mystical aspects of "centered" union. They instructed us to empty our minds of everything but sensual pleasure. "Learn to touch," they chanted. "Understand your bodies. Relax. Experience your sensations."

This was all very well, as far as it went. Yet most of us have no particular problems with our lateral spinothalamic tracts, our posterior columns, or our Herring-Breuer reflexes. We can feel and we can breathe. We experience sensation; we massage and are massaged; we appreciate the physical. We like voluptuous encounters; we enjoy touching sexual skin; we are pleased by a warm caress. What must we do when we find ourselves, even so, in sexual distress or dilemma, turned off, unexcited? Or if not quite so seriously afflicted, at least bored by the repetitious servicing of our sensuality?

The answer is almost always personal, as deeply related to our individual selves as our concepts of dignity and God. Profound response to sex, as to poetry, art, or music, lies in the emotions. I've concluded from my own life and from the accounts of those who can tap their emotions that sex is best when it contains some strong feeling: anything from great grief to great tenderness to great elation. Orgasms are most satisfying when they occur at the peak of such feelings—those that mock our mortality as well as those that affirm it.

I think a great deal about ways to help people to express themselves beyond their present limits—a few stifled moans and breathless exclamations—to stop being silent sexual robots. The researchers have groped toward this goal, too, in their own indirect fashion. Several years ago, in *Science*, investigators reported their work with the "copulatory vocalizations of chacma baboons and gibbons." One downright embarrassing finding was that baboons make more interesting and complex noises than humans do. Compared with human sonograms, the recorded baboon endearments show greater variety and intensity than human sexual communication in its presently retarded state. I'd bet they convey more meaning, too.

In the past, people were in fact capable of intricate mating sounds. In ancient India, instructions to lovers included great varieties of bird and animal imitations to express broad ranges of response. These refinements belonged to a time when man was closer to nature. I find it amusing to imagine, for a moment, that we could relearn them. We could listen to other animals and then warble, pipe, and flute at one another. On reaching orgasm, we could mightily roar, howl, trumpet, bellow. And as we did, we might at last reach our feelings. On the other hand, such mimetics today would as likely land a suitor in the booby hatch as in the boudoir. And what a pedagogical demand it would place on the sex therapist!

Comprehending our emotions during sex is difficult. Indeed, Coleridge's reply to the woman who insisted that he give her a technique for responding to poetry may be an appropriate caution. "Madam," he said, "think you nothing of itself will come, but we must do the seeking?" Feelings may surface as from some primordial abyss, or they may descend, as though from a realm above. As Coleridge pointed out, one does not order emotion, nor does one quite know where it comes from.

Sometimes, to almost everyone, it happens. In the midst of our ascending pleasure we feel a familiar constriction at the throat. Soon the warm fluid is on our cheeks. We know we are crying. If we do not make some sound, if we do not recognize the tears, the feeling will disappear into the hell or heaven or id whence it emerged. We will lose it and, along with it, any remote chance of learning what it is and why it came to us now. Are we mourning our childhood, our lost parents, our lover soon to be gone, our life soon to be ended? Are we mourning the lives—too early extinguished—of others who never experienced this love? Is it all mankind we cry for? Why should we now think such thoughts? Maybe we do not weep enough at other times. Perhaps we may think these thoughts now, and only now, because we trust our lover to comfort us against all trouble and all despair and death.

Sometimes a scream rises up at the summit of our pleasure, not a scream of pain, but of triumph, a glory that we feel. If we silence it, we may never know the barrier we have passed.

Rarely, we laugh. The gaiety fills our bellies, and we breathe it out in bursts of amazing rollicking delight—at having been born and lived to now, at being here, at having been bad and good, at cheating death—and at the notion of a world full of funny, wrinkled babies squawling to become postmen and presidents.

Drugs, Transference, and Sex

KNOWING WHAT MEDICATIONS people take is as crucial to a sex therapist as understanding whether or not they get along with their partners. I constantly run the risk of embarrassing patients' physicians because the drugs they have prescribed may so evidently cause the disorder for which they send a patient to see me. Sometimes the most innocent-seeming drugs can cause stunning side effects.

For most of us, just knowing which drugs will interfere with what sexual function is sufficient. Every day, it seems, I read or hear that still another drug has an adverse effect on sex. Indeed, nearly every drug known to have an effect on sex can cause impotence in men and some equivalent of impotence in women. Of course, one must remember that people have individual responses to drugs. What impairs one person may not trouble another. Dosage is critical, too. Some can tolerate more than others. Just as most people can take an aspirin, a cup of coffee, or a glass of wine without any trouble, so most can handle prescribed drugs without sexual side effects.

I once made a list of prescription drugs that are fairly well known to impinge on sex. I began with the drugs that doctors give for illness. I set down my notes here so that people taking drugs can check on them, but I've indented my list so that non-drug takers can easily skip to the end of it and get to what may be more interesting, the discussion of sex and the drugs used for the purpose of altering the mind, the psychoactive drugs.

Among the medications that doctors prescribe, virtually the entire spectrum of blood-pressure lowering agents may cause sexual disorder. The reactions to antihypertensives include interference with libido, erection, ejaculation, and orgasm. Not all antihypertensive drugs cause all these effects; such a symptom warrants a consultation with a physician. Some blood-pressure lowering drugs are methyl dopa (Aldomet), guanethidine (Ismelin, Esimil), reserpine (Serpasil et al.), propranolol (Inderal). Other agents include metaprolol (Lopressor), clonidine (Catapres), hydralazine (Apresoline), trimethaphan (Arfonad), and phenoxybenzamine (Dibenzyline). Doctors also control hypertension with diuretics, drugs that help reduce body water. Such drugs include the "thiazide" diuretics (Diuril, hydrochlorothiazide et al.), furosemide (Lasix), ethacrynic acid (Edecrin), and spironolactone (Aldactone). These may contribute to trouble with erection, and some may interfere with libido and ejaculation as well. Other cardiovascular agents, such as the antiarrhythmics and beta blockers, may also cause problems.

The anticholinergic medications used mainly to release bowel spasms may cause impotence and ejaculatory dysfunction. Some of these are atropine, homatropine, the belladonna alkaloids, scopolamine, and propantheline (Probanthine).

Antihistamines have been reported to interfere with erection and libido. Certain nasal decongestants as well as nonprescription cold remedies containing a combination of antihistaminic and anticholinergic drugs may impair libido, erection, and ejaculation. These effects occur only in doses much higher than those recommended. No studies have been done on the sexual consequences of long-term habituation to ordinary quantities.

The sedative-hypnotic drugs may, of course, interfere with libido. These include the barbiturates, diazepam (Valium), chlordiazepoxide (Librium), methaqualone (Quaalude), and others. The barbiturates may also interfere with erection and orgasm, and chlordiazepoxide has on one occasion been reported to interfere with ejaculation.

Drugs used to control psychosis, the phenothiazines, may have negative effects largely upon erection and ejaculation. One drug, thioridazine (Mellaril), has often been reported to affect ejaculation and orgasm; both thioridazine and chlorpromazine (Thorazine) may affect libido.

Antidepressants, the most common formerly being the "tricyclics" (Elavil, Tofranil et al.), and now the newer serotonin re-uptake inhibitors and drugs that have followed Prozac, may affect libido, erection and ejaculation, as may the monoamine oxidase inhibitors.

Hormones may have varying effects. Androgens in excess may reduce libido in men. Estrogens, given to men to control certain forms of cancer, may reduce their sexual ability. Progestational agents may reduce female libido.

Many miscellaneous drugs, like digitalis, used for severe conditions, may cause erectile difficulties. Lithium and disulfuram (Antabuse) may also interfere with erection.

The drugs mentioned above merely suggest the immense number of agents that can cause sexual problems. If a person takes any drug at all and suffers a sexual problem soon after, he or she ought to consult a physician to see if the drug is responsible.

The second category of drugs is composed of the weeds, powders, liquids, pellets, and potions that people imbibe, inject, inhale, or swallow to alter the functions of their mind and body for nontherapeutic purposes. In excess, they can all cause impotence. They may also cause other sexual problems. Some users, however, claim vast sexual benefits from "recreational" drugs. Medicine insists that there is no true aphrodisiac among them, yet the popularity of drugs like cocaine and the amphetamines owes a great deal to their sexual effects. The pharmacological establishment remains firm in its view that one cannot demonstrate a consistent and direct line of sexual stimulation. I believe that the establishment is correct. As opposed to the direct effects, however, the indirect effects of drugs on sexuality seem intriguing. Why does a particular drug stimulate sexual feelings in some people but not in others?

The recreational drugs are "psychomimetic"—that is, they mimic our psyches, our ego states. Many of them give some people a sense of comfort, a feeling of safety, a sense of blocking out danger. In thinking about these drugs I've gradually evolved the concept that the various drug-induced states of mind, starting with comfort or satiety, may be sexually stimulating in an indirect fashion.

There are three classes of drugs most commonly taken for their psychomimetic effects: the hypno-sedatives, or sleep-inducing drugs (downers), the hallucinogens, and the stimulants (uppers). One of the most fascinating aspects of all this is the way the "sedative" drugs may take a person along the route to sexual pleasure without directly activating any sexual center.

The barbiturates depress the life-promoting activities of sensitive tissues, especially the central nervous system. We don't know how they do it, but they contribute to reducing anxiety. They slow down the brain. Our brain cells appear to use less oxygen and to work less effectively when under their influence. Barbiturates can cause anything from mild sedation to coma.

Feeling sedated or sleepy—incapable of performing complex actions, the way we are when our brains are not functioning correctly—has different effects on different people. Some resent being in the power of an outside force that takes away their control. Most of us, indeed, would dislike imposing this much powerlessness on ourselves, especially if we are alert, awake, and functional. Users, however, experience the initial barbiturate effect as pleasantly calming, taking matters out of their hands. They can't function too well; therefore, why try? It is satisfying, comforting even, to be out of the struggle. "Nodding out" may be a kind of satiety, like a baby falling asleep when it is full. As suggested by Dr. William Frosch in an early paper on this subject, it may also serve to block out unpleasant thoughts and feelings. We may take drugs to "knock ourselves out," or screen out the difficulties of reality. Analytically, enjoying this state is a "regressive" phenomenon, a return to a babyhood time when our brains were not so well developed, our motor-coordination not so keen, our thought processes less available to us. We associate this state with being taken care of. The drug recapitulates babyhood and puts us in a condition of dependent somnolence.

In the analytic condition known as "transference," we superimpose the feelings we had in old relationships onto new ones. Thus, dependent feelings toward an analyst frequently resemble those toward a parent. In some mysterious way, those experiencing dependent feelings often also experience sexual arousal. That is why so many people "fall in love" with their analysts. This arousal has been the subject of much inquiry as to whether or not it is "appropriate." Proper or not, "resistance" or not, it often happens. The analytic situation is not the only circumstance in which it occurs. Any authority figure who rouses dependent feelings may stimulate sexual feelings along with them. Teachers, doctors, and priests most commonly elicit them.

A "positive transference," with or without sexual feelings, exists when a person believes the authority can, does, or will satisfy these desires. It may promote excellent and productive relations, if the dependency is appropriate. Mutually acceptable reliance, with an exchange of warm feeling, is one of the most delightful conditions granted human beings to experience.

("Negative transference" commonly refers to the feelings of rage, pain, and abandonment when one believes that the authority figure is incapable of or unwilling to give this support. Adults may repeatedly make neurotic errors, sometimes fully knowing that they are doing so, by depending on the wrong people. For this, we may experience intense shame. We may also make neurotic mistakes by failing to depend on trustworthy people.)

The point is that the pill that makes a person sleepy may come to represent a pleasurably dependent, regressive state of mind that can lead—as mysteriously as the transference phenomenon in psychoanalysis often leads—to sexual arousal or receptivity. Sex is safe. One is not in control. Protection is imagined, anxiety dispelled, inhibitions loosened in the jumble that the drug makes of our nervous system.

Similar effects occur with the popular methaqualone, also known as Quaalude. An even pleasanter sedation may be experienced with small quantities of opium and its congeners: morphine, heroin, codeine, and the like. In addition to inducing quiescence, they may alter perception of pain so that all the normal aches we experience may be reduced. These drugs mimic exactly those recently discovered natural body compounds, the enkephalins and endorphins, so responsible for our experience of pain and pleasure. The opioids have been called "God's own medicine." It is extraordinary that the creator of life chose to place compounds almost precisely like those so important to human well-being in the juices of the poppy seed.

For those to whom feelings of relaxation and contentment are helpful (as well as those who may wish chemical assistance in delaying orgasm and ejaculation), very small quantities of opium or opium derivatives may be pleasantly erotic.

It is important to note here that I am not talking of drug addiction, of the "orgasmic rush" users describe on mainlining heroin, or of the sensual fantasies without the interest in sexual activity that chronic or heavy opioid use may create. I am talking about social narcotic use in a preaddictive phase, probably seen more often a century ago than today. By the same token, I am not discussing barbiturate addiction: the "downer high" that comes after a heavy dose has worn off, the irritable phases, the periods of sheer disorientation. At this level of both barbiturate and narcotic abuse, the erotic often matters no longer. People regress to entirely infantile, pregenital styles.

The next group of psychoactive drugs are called "psychedelic" or "psychotomimetic." Loosely speaking, this means that they make us crazy. In pharmacological language, they "provide a drug model of psychosis." When psychedelics are working to produce a benign madness, it may be said that they create an ego state known as "fusion." In psychiatric jargon, fusion means that a person's "boundaries" become "fluid." At one level, this means that the senses are confused and disturbed; most commonly auditory experiences are transformed into visual ones. Noise creates kaleidoscopic visual effects. Music may be visible as color or seem to float through the air like blips on an oscilloscope. Vision may be distorted as well: The normal may appear either exceptionally beautiful or keenly grotesque. Perceptions of time, space, and motion—the relative phenomena—are no longer tied to our usual earthly landmarks. An LSD trip represents a journey into worlds outside our Newtonian reality, into that cosmic territory where, they say, the body becomes one with time, space, motion, color, sound, and—most important—other people.

Analysts consider this, too, a regressive state of mind. They recall to us those periods when a pregnant mother cannot tell the difference between her own body and that of her embryonic child, and they describe how long it takes before a child's developing mind can distinguish between its own body and that of its mother. Many years are required for the separation to take place fully. A baby probably experiences that it is still part of the mother when its cry of hunger is satisfied by the breast. During later times of sorting out reality, all kinds of fears, confusions, and charming childish beliefs are possible: Do objects speak? Can magic happen? Does the boogeyman live in the closet? We need a light at night to make sure that our belongings do not assume fantastic shapes. In my generation, we read fairy tales because in them snow maidens turned to queens. We almost believed, too, that Batman, Robin, Superman, and Wonder Woman existed. The child combines and fuses images with reality, using that capacity we call imagination, a gift necessary for sorting out the nuances of experience.

In the adult transference, a sense of desiring fusion is a powerful motive for "love." As adults, we experience this as identification, or a wish for close emotional involvement. Little in life can seem so exhilarating as becoming part of someone else or allowing them to become part of you. Some people are even capable of an ecstasy of fusion with a beloved; musicians, I think, are most comfortable in this state, for to them the emotion may be synonymous with musical sound. Take this description of lovemaking by Georges Julien Ohm, a presumably musical French psychologist, for example:

> Above all, it would be impossible for me to differentiate myself from my partner. . . . That stream of consciousness which I have become is a hypersensitivity of my skin, my eyes, my tongue. It is as though awareness were made flesh. . . . The best analogy is provided by music. When I am completely absorbed in listening to a piece of music, I cease to exist, at least in the psychologic sense of a different self, i.e., a differential entity. I am one with the music. At the equivalent stage in lovemaking, I am one with the various sensations. My body is not merely alive, it has become "electric."

Compare this with Timothy Leary's psychedelic experience as described in *Playboy* in 1966:

> Ordinarily, sexual communication involves one's own chemicals, pressure and interactions of a very localized nature—in what the psychologists call the erogenous zones. A vulgar, dirty concept, I think. When you're making love under LSD, it's as though every cell in your body—and you have trillions—is making love with every cell in her body. Your hand doesn't caress her skin but sinks down into and merges with ancient dynamos of ecstasy within her. . . . Merging, yielding, flowing union, communion. It's all lovemaking. You make love with candlelight, with sound waves from a record player, with a bowl of fruit on the table, with the trees. You're in pulsating harmony with all the energy around you.

Again, the chemical that one ingests can simulate the feeling one once had with a parent, now translated into sexual arousal and making love. Fusion with the mother becomes fusion with the pill, which then inspires fusion with a lover. The psychedelic erotic experience, when it occurs, may be the most powerful of all. Some people, incapable of fusion without the drug, may seek their best—and even most religious—feelings in powdered form. They cannot feel these emotions without the magic potion.

LSD is not uniformly an inspiration to lovers' bliss, however. Having taken my medical training in the sixties, I had ample opportunity to spend many long emergency room nights bringing people out of bad trips. Still, people keep on risking permanent impairment of their sanity to have feelings that can be experienced without drugs by the commonest person capable of transcending ordinary boundaries and truly making love.

As for the stimulants, they rev us up. They are called "sympathomimetic" drugs because they imitate the activating effects of the sympathetic nervous system. Both the natural and the synthetic stimulants increase the use of our body fuels, excite our hearts, increase our breathing rate, reduce our appetite, and keep us vigorously awake. Takers of amphetamines, methedrine, cocaine, and other "uppers" are not satisfied by their own natural stimulants, such as epinephrine and norepinephrine. Normally, they may live in a dull, depressed state; they may feel lethargic and useless. The drug helps them to feel the excitement that they would experience simply at being alive if they were emotionally complete. Indeed, stimulants may take a person beyond even normal euphoria, to sensations of masterful triumph, as most of us are aware.

In the transference, these feelings may be likened to those when a baby takes its first successful steps, speaks its first words, or masters any other functions that have been labeled "propriate." When we walk, run, write, read, add a column correctly, learn to ski, skate, or drive a car, we are accomplishing propriate functions. Early on, our parents attended our first triumphs and were proud of us. Whenever we accomplish something new, we may, at some level, be reliving those moments in which they safely accompanied us through the hazards of learning and loved us for our achievement.

In the mysterious fashion of transferential feelings, mastery may encourage a person's sexuality. We have a great libidinal hunger always waiting to be satisfied; we may seize the opportunities of triumph to enjoy our celebration feasts.

Amphetamines make some people feel very good without having achieved anything at all, even the allegedly simple feat of remaining contentedly alive. For them, the drug provides the self-satisfaction that admiring parents can impart. People get "high." Often they seek to return again and again to this state and soon burn themselves out, lapsing into impotence, ejaculatory disturbance, and orgasmic failure, not to mention depression of psychotic dimensions. Nevertheless, the drug provides great numbers of people with such a vigor and enthusiasm for life, however temporary, that we can hardly condemn them for seeking it out. They seem not to know that there are other ways to feel better.

Alcohol and marijuana are more complicated social drugs. They are capable of producing more than one effect, which may vary a great deal even within a single person, according to mood, circumstance, and dose. Alcohol is basically a depressant, though initially it may create a euphoria that appears related more to acceptance of impaired function than to mastery. "I can do whatever I want," says the drinker, "and it's okay because I'm high." Later on, the basic satiation-sleep-dependency syndrome sets in, as a person becomes more and more intoxicated. The psychic confusion of drunkenness may also somewhat resemble a psychedelic experience.

Marijuana may have sedative, psychedelic, and stimulant effects, too, again depending on dose, circumstance, and a person's mood set.

Since both of these drugs are so variable in their ability to create satiety, fusion, or activation effects, we may expect that they are associated with sexual arousal—in small doses—more often than the other drugs. They have more effects that lead to sexuality. That appears to be the case.

These two social drugs—alcohol and marijuana—I might add, may interfere with sexual function, impairing libido, erection, ejaculation, and orgasm. So can the narcotics—heroin, morphine, all the opioids—and the stimulants such as the amphetamines and cocaine.

Drugs are a frequent topic in conversations with my patients. They have become a factor in sexuality that they were not when I started practice. But today people aren't as giddy and uncritical about drugs as they have been; they know about the snake in that particular Eden. Yet they dream of the perfect drug, the magical sex facilitator. They are desperate to be vulnerable, willing to buy the devil's powders and to pay a great price in order to be human.

The Theory and Practice of Anal Sex

JUST AS WE may be trained not to think of our bottoms as
seats of pleasure, so we may be trained to enjoy them. Medically
speaking, the ano-rectum has the potential for being as effective
a conduit for sexual sensation as the vagina or the penis. Many
of its sensations may be the same as—I have heard some say
greater than—those conveyed by the routine genitals. Supplied
by the same nerves, contracting during orgasm at the same time
that the vaginal muscles, the uterus, the urinary sphincter, and
the muscles of the male pelvic floor contract, related spatially to
those organs, and covered by a "sexual skin," the anus could be
experienced purely sexually were it not for its function of controlling the elimination of waste.

I believe that the mind alone keeps the anus (and buttocks,
too, in some cases) out of the sexual province. It might also be
said that the mind alone allows anal intercourse to be a sexual
act. The brain's control over sexual sensitivity dominates with
great precision in this area. Only the psyche's influence on the
body could explain why some people experience extraordinarily

intense pleasure through anal eroticism, while others can't understand how anyone could possibly enjoy anything associated with defecation. Today, of course, the association of anal sex with AIDS, acquired through damaged or bleeding rectal structures, has made the practice more taboo than ever. Still, among monogamous partners and those with special physical disabilities, the practice continues in a high enough percentage of the population to merit compassionate discussion.

Sometimes couples come for sex therapy because one or the other partner has been physically damaged. Trauma to vaginal nerve supply, while rare, does occur in childbirth and other surgery. One patient lost her ability for normal sensation after being dilated to increase the easy flow of her menses. Another had a difficult hysterectomy that resulted in the creation of a very short vagina, which could contain only the head of her husband's penis. Both women sought sex therapy. A man who had had his entire penis removed due to malignancy became my patient because he wished for some form of sexual pleasure. Another man had lost the use of his penis through an accidental "fracture" or hemorrhage in the shaft, and a third had a "micropenis," which afforded him much embarrassment and little voluptuousness. Penile implants and reconstructive surgery were either not possible or not available at the time these men consulted me. It seemed to some that anal sex could significantly assist their enjoyment of erotic life. It was an alternative to be mentioned to others. To those who were receptive I gave as much advice and encouragement as I could. I dropped the subject with those who could not tolerate it.

I teach such people to enjoy receiving anal pleasure in much the same way that I sometimes help willing people to experience other sexual arousal—by conditioning. When women have no sensation in their nipples, for example, I may suggest that they have an erotic fantasy during nipple stimulation and thus incorporate their breasts into erotic life. Similar fantasy may be used to incorporate the ano-rectum.

In some, these transitions are remarkably quick, requiring only suggestion and permission. Others, as I have said, cannot accept anal sex as a human activity, or find it difficult to alter their psyche in favor of it. Women concerned with female liberation who consider it politically demeaning to fellate a man often also think it humiliating to offer up a bottom to male delight. To them, the act is an unpleasant submission to male aggression. Those who feel this way generally cannot be persuaded otherwise. In sex, all people have their own truth.

And then there are those who believe in the inferiority of buttocks. They point out that women's "asses" have been the object of crude jokes, slaps, whistles, and patronizing pats since well before construction workers ever looked up from their sidewalk lunches to watch a woman pass. They cannot understand or respect the dignity of the human body in all its parts.

Beyond politics, there are women who have previously been hurt by untutored attempts to penetrate their rectums.

Rectal dilation is often a slow task, requiring as much patience as readying a vagina for intercourse, if not more. The quick "buttering up" that Marlon Brando did in *Last Tango in Paris* is nothing to the point. Just as a woman's vagina may suddenly dry and reject intrusion, so the anal sphincter opens and closes unexpectedly, depending on stimulation and mental set. For the inexperienced, extravagant amounts of Vaseline or K-Y jelly, and much time spent entering with a slowly rotating finger, are necessary. For women, simultaneous clitoral stimulation is also an exciting and distracting stimulus. For some women a vagino-rectal massage—thumb in rectum and fingers in vagina, or vice versa—plus clitoral stimulation can also be thrilling. The rectal vibrator or dildo may contribute, too, to anal eroticism in both men and women. But one must be careful never to use an instrument that can slip into the rectum accidentally. These tend to travel upward through the colon. Abdominal surgery has to be performed occasionally to remove such vibrators, some still buzzing, from deep within the bowel.

I don't believe that studies have been done on "normal" anorectal reaction to sexual excitement. I have heard it said that the anus of a rectally experienced homosexual male opens receptively by itself when he is aroused. That, in fact, is supposed to be a clue to detecting the homosexual male. I wonder if experience is really necessary for rectal reaction. Do some people, men and women, dilate rectally on excitement while others don't, more as a matter of physiology than psychology? Certainly one has to be positively disposed, but given that, can all people do it? I have had female patients whose backgrounds one would expect to have made anal sex unthinkable, yet they blandly admit that "of course" they like anal sex, and "have it all the time." Some women feel that they can never enjoy anal sex because their sphincters are too tight, or because they have been traumatized by a man too eager to push his way in.

Men sometimes have trouble learning anal sex because they often associate it so strongly with homosexuality. They may or may not be able to resolve their feelings or accept an accompanying fantasy. In my practice men seem to have less difficulty than women with being on the receiving end of anal pleasure. Perhaps this is because stimulation of the prostate gland occurs anally and is more directly exciting than most sensations women can respond to in the same area.

I often encounter the problem couple where the man presses for anal sex and his partner rejects it. This may lead to a dissatisfaction on both sides that pervades the marriage and is symbolic of other problems. Occasionally, a woman wants to receive it, but her partner finds the task repulsive. If the couple can achieve intimate sexual pleasure by other means, I do not take it upon myself to insist that one partner's whim be satisfied. That would be helping one person to dominate another. But if a man or woman should sincerely wish to overcome guilt or reluctance, then I am willing to help.

Many women enjoy anal sex because it is truly easier for them. They need hardly exert themselves. Yet contrary to popular opinion, anal sex need not be at all passive. Different movements are possible, depending on whether one lies prone, kneels, or sits. Eliminating the need to worry about pregnancy also helps some women to enjoy it. There are many caveats, however. One patient who came to me with his wife for other reasons described a lifelong pattern of vaginal intercourse followed by anal insertion for ejaculation. Since the movement was from vagina to anus, there was no need to wash between. He was pleased that an intercourse with simultaneous orgasm was possible at any time. In reality, this practice was not without serious risk of both conception and male infection.

Whether or not people who have no special requirement should learn to enjoy anal sex is a question often asked. Like whether or not to have an affair, it is a question no one but the owner of the body can answer. I can suggest that if people do not have an easy affinity for anal activity—if they don't enjoy their bowels or are constantly upset by one or another gastrointestinal complaint—they may have to overcome too many inhibitions to achieve sensual return. Situations where trauma has occurred, or where childbirth has left a wide introitus or a loose vagina, however, may encourage some to a trial of anal sex.

It is important to remember that, above and beyond HIV infection, there are several medical dangers to anal intercourse. Men may acquire infections of the urethra and bladder through the passage of coliform and other bacteria; women may acquire vaginal infections if there has been no cleansing of the penis between its contact with fecal material and with the vagina.

Although the rectum is normally empty enough to contain a penis without direct contact with feces, it is still a contaminated area. A condom should always be used, although the sex manuals of yesteryear advised a thorough penile scrubbing before entering a vagina after anal sex. In the ill-advised event that a condom is not used, certainly a good wash, including a cleansing of the male urethral opening with mushy soap, should be performed after anal sex, even if intercourse doesn't follow.

Mechanical trauma—fissures, hemorrhoids, and other damage—may also occur. The anus was not designed for intercourse. Great caution is practical.

Strong opinions are held about the pros and cons of anal sex. A vigorous conservative segment maintains that the practice of gaining sexual pleasure through any contact at all with the anus, whether that aperture belongs to oneself or anyone else, constitutes a perversion. They feel that the colon and the sphincter should serve only the function of elimination. On the other side of the controversy are those who feel that in anal sex a person is stimulated as no other manner allows. They suggest men are extraordinarily excited by the snug fit of the anal muscles and the round, full pressure of receptive buttocks, while women are thrilled by the singular intimacy and trust, and the daring. It was no accident of nature, they say, that made anal sex a workable alternative to procreative coupling.

Probably neither faction reasons fully. Our bodies, our training, and our character determine what we will enjoy and what we will reject. Our psyches, partly inherited, partly conditioned, and partly independent, create the emotion that determines the act's significance. What one person does with care and tenderness, another may enact with coldness or brutality. Emotional overtones accompany virtually all behaviors; by these we judge their propriety. Provided that harm is neither inflicted nor intended, all forms of human sexuality possess intrinsic goodness.

On Cunnilingus

SOME YEARS AGO I realized I wasn't sure of the precise derivation of *cunnilingus*, so I went to the big Webster's dictionary that I bought in 1960. I hoped that Noah Webster's intellectual descendants had heard of it. They had. The translation from the Latin cuts the nonsense with eloquent precision. "Cunni-" derives from *cunnus*, meaning "vulva," and "lingus" stems from *lingere*, "to lick." Cunnilingus is the art of licking the vulva. The scholars who Latinized English did not equivocate, although they added a certain medieval mystery to common practice.

Licking the vulva, or any other part of the female reproductive anatomy, was considered bad form in America until half a century ago. I can remember that it was only after Dr. Theodoor H. Van DeVelde, in his book *Ideal Marriage*, pronounced it an acceptable way to arouse and lubricate a woman, that the people of my generation began to try it more. I'm sure there were other equally important figures who wrote the same sort of things, but among my contemporaries his blessing and sanction gave married couples the impetus to treat each other more like people and

211

less like reproductive machines. Men began to pay more attention to women's clitorises, and women began to feel entitled to pleasure.

Indeed, in response to societal permission for oral sex, the public began to idealize it. I have even heard some claims that most women prefer cunnilingus to intercourse and would select it over other forms of lovemaking. What makes cunnilingus particularly pleasurable? Why are some of us ecstatic about it while others abhor it?

Many people have told me the fantasy that cunnilingus was originally a lesbian art that heterosexuals have only recently begun to learn. They suspect that lesbians are the only ones who really know how to do it. Certain lesbians may be virtuosos, but actually many are not intuitively inspired or more informed than men. I've found that they frequently need as much instruction as heterosexuals do. Much of the commentary to follow may be interpreted as referring to both lesbian and heterosexual relationships.

Enjoying cunnilingus most essentially involves the concept of the genital kiss. Oral lips meet genital lips, and an active communication begins. A woman can use her sphincter muscles to meet and match a man's kiss, just as she might respond to him with her mouth. The person performing cunnilingus should be familiar with a partner's visible genital expression, her stages of excitement. He should recognize the rosy open fullness of a woman's genital lips when she is excited and appreciate the acceleration of her muscular tensions. No other form of lovemaking affords such opportunity for understanding and controlling a woman's approaches to orgasm.

Combined cunnilingus and finger-stroking may be immensely exciting. Dual stimulation encourages multiple climaxes in those who are sensitive. It may also please those who like externally induced orgasms as a warm-up and prelude to intercourse. With an easily orgasmic partner, eliminating clitoral stimulation as she nears climax, or stopping entirely for a few seconds, will help to prolong the pleasure. The art of stimulation to high excitement followed by deep thrusting of penis or dildo can sometimes induce orgasms that last for minutes rather than seconds, each contraction emerging slowly and deeply rather than in rapid superficial sequence.

The varieties of sexual pleasure that people may technically give one another are amply described in our already overwhelming sexual archive. For me as a sex therapist, the most challenging concerns are the barriers to pleasure. A simple but major obstacle to the joy of oral sex is that not everyone means the same thing by cunnilingus. Just as some consider that fellatio involves licking the tip of a man's penis while massaging the rest of it manually, and others feel that the full Latin impact of the word implies a sword-swallower's ability to take a penis deep in the throat, past the point of being able to breathe, so interpretations of cunnilingus differ. Some think it is licking the clitoris. Others think it means inserting the tongue like a penis. Still others feel it refers to an all-around wash, including anal stroking and stimulation.

For those who can appreciate many varieties of pleasure, oral love implies all of the above and more. Good kissing also includes proper sucking, mainly of the clitoris and vulva. The use of hands, lips, and tongue, nose and chin, hair and forehead, of blowing and breathing rhythms, and even of deep vocal vibrations, may become part of a lover's repertoire. (Men must be warned that it is dangerous to blow directly into a woman's vagina; it can create an air bubble that may find its way into her bloodstream or body cavities and kill her.) The woman, too, can assist cunnilingus. She can guide a man's head to where she would like it, spread her legs and move her hips to enhance or suggest her lover's head and tongue movement, or kneel and bring her vagina down upon her partner's mouth to stimulate herself or him. She may use her own hands to augment his activity. The couple may try moderately gymnastic positions to bring the vulva closer to the partner's face without causing neckstrain, such as lying head down over the back of an easy chair or using pillows to elevate the buttocks and make access easier in bed.

In any event, the woman who likes having her clitoris stimulated with gentle, even, regular movements means something different by cunnilingus than the one who most enjoys having a broad, strong tongue caressing her thighs and vagina.

When couples come for sex therapy, women's inability to tell their lovers precisely what they like creates a major problem. And even if told properly where and how, many men continue to have such an imperfect sense of female anatomy that they often lose their way. In addition, certain men simply cannot fulfill their partners' desires. Occasionally it takes sex therapy to discover that nature has given them a small tongue, or one whose movement is hampered by a tight frenulum—the strip of flesh connecting the underside of the tongue to the base of the mouth. Some of these men choose to have a frenectomy, the removal or splitting of this band, to free their lingual movement and satisfy their mates!

Thus while cunnilingus has been vastly popularized as a joyous and rewarding activity, it continues to require sophisticated information and more accurate communication than many people are able to achieve. The number of unsatisfied women who move their lover's head away from their genitals and start intercourse before they are ready, simply because the oral-genital contact has not been what they wanted, probably far exceeds the number of the satisfied. In theory they may like oral sex a great deal. In fact, a proficient lover—one who can understand their preferences—may be hard to find.

Today this paucity has become a political issue. As women feel deserving of more sexual attention, they feel rejected and demeaned when they do not receive it. Many become hostile toward men who do not perform cunnilingus, or who do it poorly or without pleasure. Indeed, when power politics enter the bedroom, no issue flames so rapidly as oral sex.

Many men cannot accept the practice as a political issue, however. They love their wives and would provide them with every service and equality, but they do not enjoy cunnilingus. They are either repelled by it or phobic of it. Helping them often becomes a task of the sex therapist. In dysfunctions that seem at first to be orgasmic disorders, the hidden agenda frequently concerns a husband's fears of oral sex.

At the most elementary level, many men find female genital odor unpleasant and are afraid to say so. Their fears are often justified, for few criticisms can offend women as readily as being told that their odor is unpleasant. One woman, whose husband mentioned lightly that her aroma was a bit strong, never again allowed him to have oral sex with her. Since this was the only way she could reach orgasm, it meant that she refrained from orgasm with her husband for ten years. Another dwelt in the misery of what she suspected might be a loveless marriage because her husband hadn't the courage to ask her to wash. Some gynecologists perpetuate such disasters by telling women that it is best for their vaginal health not to douche. This may be true for a sexually inactive woman. Women who frequently have intercourse, and whose vaginas are inhabited by menstrual remnants, spermatic fluid, spermicide or lubricant, and the bacteria of oral and digital manipulation, need occasionally to refresh their sexual passages. A sex therapist may reveal this problem tactfully and suggest a healthy regimen.

Men do have obstacles to oral pleasure that go beyond considerations such as scent or know-how. After all, the male mechanic by hobby or profession who can locate and repair complicated circuits or do ingenious woodworking should really have little trouble identifying a few major organs and doing some simple digital or lingual exercises. The fact is that anxieties about physical techniques often reflect deeply rooted psychological troubles.

Some of the psychological barriers are much like those in fellatio. Many men feel unduly humbled by the nether position, especially if they are called on to kneel. They don't want to kiss anyone's bottom parts. Other, even more insecure men cannot give anything at all to sex, any physical effort, without feeling used.

A significant barrier to male pleasure in cunnilingus is a phenomenon known as castration anxiety. Troubled males afflicted by fears of injury feel vaguely uneasy confronting a woman's vagina; they experience a sense of deformity, or something missing. They don't like to look closely at the place and are particularly put off by menstrual blood, as though it denoted a wound. They may perform with grim stoicism, or maybe not at all. One man I treated recounted fantasies of a vagina as a bloody, mutilated space where a penis ought to grow. Another, afraid that his wife's vagina wanted to possess his penis, had to be trained slowly to look, to touch, to feel.

One of the most helpful techniques I have used to help men overcome castration anxiety (and to help certain women deal with penis envy as well) has been to explain the anatomy of the female genitalia in penile terms. The vulva or vaginal lips are embryologically equivalent to the scrotum. (The woman's equivalents of testicles, the ovaries, are protected by their placement deep inside.) The long back-to-front area of the large vaginal lips may also be thought of as something like the shaft of a penis, with spongy chambers (also placed deeply within) that fill with blood. If one imagines the penis divided in half with erectile chambers on either side, one can relate stroking the vulva to stimulating the shaft of the penis. At the summit of the vulva is the clitoris, of which only the tip, like the tip of an iceberg, shows. Most people are familiar with the analogy of the clitoris to the glans penis.

In a sense, a woman has an organ very much like a penis that fills, engorges, and forms a palpable mass between her legs when she is excited. She also, of course, has the additional bounty of a vagina, cervix, and uterus, which contribute their unique sensations. Some women, when not feeling ovulation pain, claim that they can detect the pleasure of having their ovaries indirectly stroked on intercourse, and others are aware of their womb being caressed on intercourse and on deep abdominal massage.

Somehow, when men visualize the vulva and clitoris as a kind of erect penis between a woman's legs, a great deal of castration anxiety is relieved. This concept has often been enough to help many men, particularly those with either overt or covert homosexual trends, to perform cunnilingus.

The common notion that oral sex with a woman is like eating a good meal—or enjoying the interior of a ripe melon, full face to the core on a hot summer day—may be appealing to the lusty but does not generally help the phobic or the timid. As a sex therapist, I have also had little success with berry-flavored douches or whipped cream toppings as incitements to gustatory experiment. Most troubled men cannot proceed so dramatically. The analogy of eating stirs castration anxiety too strongly.

Timid or phobic men must first be taught to look, to identify parts, to touch and know what they are touching. Most important is not to expect to experience pleasure. At first, tolerance of distress is all a therapist can ask. Usually, after a short time of touching and feeling, anxiety diminishes and disappears. The same holds true of first growing accustomed to smelling and sniffing, and then touching with lips, and finally with tongue. Pleasure through the use of unrelated fantasy or music may help to distract and relieve the anxiety. Pleasure in the act itself may come along later—much later—after repeated feedback from the woman's enjoyment and with the satisfaction of possessing a powerful new skill.

One may note here that "69," the celebrated practice of simultaneous fellatio and cunnilingus, does not generally assist the fearful. Giving and receiving at the same time tend to distract from pleasure and increase anxiety about performance. It is difficult to focus on receiving pleasure while one is thinking about giving it and wondering about the effect. Even sophisticates have difficulty in achieving mutual pleasure in this art until they are so familiar with each other's preferences that they don't have to think much about what they are doing. Novices had best take turns.

Women may be as inhibited as men in the practice of cunnilingus. Many cannot accept it because they do not feel worthy of so much flattering attention. Women's sense of their own unworthiness both causes and results from poor sexual relations. Compared to most women, men are genital exhibitionists. Even shy men generally have far less trouble being seen than women, who tend to prefer darkness to light, eyes closed to eyes open. They often hardly move while being stimulated. To be watched is to be criticized. Self-conscious about how long it may take them to have orgasm, they prematurely stop allowing themselves pleasure. A mere wisp of genital odor and they worry about offending male sensitivity. Or they feel selfish because they think men want only the "real thing"—intercourse. Learning to feel good and worthy enough to receive oral love in queenly estate often requires more than simple permission or relief of guilt. It may involve doing over one's entire self-image.

Many men become superb oral lovers because they want to make up for having problems with potency or ejaculation. Just as it may in part be true that "flat-chested women work harder," so it is true that many men, aware of their deficits, build up their skills.

As in all of life, no matter how worthwhile the outcome, there are risks. Men's mouths may transmit infections to women's vaginas, which may likewise deliver organisms to mouths. The AIDS virus may be present, although in reduced concentrations compared to blood and semen, in saliva and other body fluids. Promiscuous "wet" sex is not an option.

Even with trusted partners, one should be careful of herpetic "cold sores." (A person should not make love when he or she has one that is open, visible, or palpable.) In the '70's, as couples became more experimental, even syphilitic chancres appeared in curious places—on the lips and ears, for example. I advised choosing one's playmates carefully then, although it was not the trend; now I suggest even more meticulously taking no risk of AIDS by mating as monogamously as possible.

Still, in ever increasing numbers, as best I can tell, women are asking their mates to attempt cunnilingus. No law has been written to the effect that "thou shalt enjoy oral sex"; indeed, the laws against it are gradually being removed from the books. Like many social pleasures—conversation, sports, scotch and soda—it takes some practice and getting used to. Certainly the pleasure seems worth the effort.

As women's images of themselves improve, their opinion of the beauty of their sex organs should also improve, and they will be likely to enjoy cunnilingus more. They may ever more blithely utter those heartfelt, age-old requests: "Up a little higher" and "Down a little lower."

Postcoital Feelings

WHEN MY HUSBAND and I were first married, we didn't have jobs. We thought we were going to become famous writers when we grew up (he was twenty-two and I was nineteen). So we made love a lot, often for two and three days at a time. Writers were supposed to make love in order to have something to write about, I used to believe. I suppose I still do.

Even though it was difficult in those days to distinguish between pre- and postcoital moments, I do remember that he used to feel abandoned between climaxes, when I would want to rest quietly for a while, and he would want to chat, smoke, eat, and amuse me. He was utterly charming and he did a great imitation of a llama to get my attention, but to no avail. I was pensive. He was social.

He would sometimes accuse me of being heartless. "You actually roll over and go to sleep!" he would say. "Just like the legendary man." Imagine—I, who had been with him for the past forty-eight hours, and doing unspeakable female things! "I need to close my eyes and think for a while, that's all," I would reply. "Besides, I like to be held while I'm sleeping. That's not like a man."

"You go to sleep like the man, and I feel left behind, like the woman," he would insist.

"You don't look like a woman," I would say, and pretty soon we'd be making love again.

People are not always content after sex. Frequently they don't merge in a haze of blissful tranquility that lasts until the next encounter. They have characterological differences, serious or not, that affect both the way they have sex and what they do afterward. I don't have to analyze the little scene between my husband and myself. In it are the seeds of all our subsequent joys and heartbreaks. Through it, I think one can detect the love, the humor, and the strain that arise from our very different natures. We have sharply contrasting personality styles that make life both difficult and wonderful.

The troubles people have during sex cause them to flounder about the bed after sex in various degrees of unrest. Many couples fail to discuss their immediate reactions to sexual dilemmas. While these need not be dissected immediately like a cadaver on the postcoital bed, they can be touched on delicately. In any case, it's well to discuss them sometime between one lovemaking experience and the next. What always amazes me is that major differences in the ways people like to make love may go unexpressed for years, even a lifetime. More people than one might imagine feel sad, isolated, frustrated, or angry after sex. They are unhappy with what has just occurred. One demure art history major was always frustrated after sex because she wanted an intensely erotic experience with a dominating man who would "talk dirty" and really "have a good time." Her husband, perfectly capable of this behavior, always treated her like porcelain because she had never hinted at her lusty inclinations. Indeed, he virtually suffered impotence from the restraint.

Even if sex has been a total delight, lovers' behavior in the postcoital period can ruin it. Many men crave earthy sexual praise and appreciation from their wives, but feel that their wives are too well bred to talk or act "that way."

The tender versus the aggressive style, pornography versus romance, drama versus deeply felt but nondemonstrative passion, activity versus passivity—these innately differing approaches make lovemaking as much of an arena, for some, as any ancient coliseum. Yet the contestants say nothing. People can keep this sort of thing to themselves forever, suppressing it until it emerges as a tic or a tryst or an unprovoked argument about the grocery bill.

Almost everyone is eager to know what his or her lover prefers, and how precisely to please, yet few ask, and few of the unsatisfied answer for fear of disturbing their partner's self-esteem, or their own. "How can I, at my age, teach this dignified woman how to stimulate me with her mouth? Has it come to this, that I need help?" "If I told him he was too rough on my clitoris, I know he'd stop altogether." "She (he) barely touches me. But I'm afraid if I ask her why, I'll be put down for something that I can't correct."

This lack of communication may be the most common cause of dissatisfaction after intercourse. One female patient felt enraged and humiliated by the sexual behavior of the last three men in her life, all of whom she considered otherwise quite attractive and pleasant. One withdrew partially during ejaculation so that she could not feel the pulsating orgasm that she enjoyed more than the thrusting. Another man seemed unwilling to allow her to have orgasms after he ejaculated, which was when she usually went on to sequential orgasms. A third was so concerned about providing her with adequate foreplay that he seemed to have little energy left to satisfy her on intercourse. Rather than confront any of them, she broke up the relationships in silent rage, inexplicable to her partners.

Men, too, may fail to tell what they like and so unwittingly destroy potentially good sexual relations. One male patient gained particular pleasure from watching and feeling a woman come to orgasm without being inside her. He liked to stimulate his partner's clitoris, observe her sex flush, touch the fine sweat that emerged on her body, experience her increased pulse rate, and look at the ebb and flow of her vaginal excitement as she approached and consummated orgasm. Although he never made this desire specifically known, he was on the verge of rejecting two women for what he thought was incompatibility with his keen visual interest. One turned out the lights and he thought she preferred the dark. Another had told him that she "liked it a different way" when he stimulated her clitoris, and he assumed she didn't care for the activity that would allow him to observe her. On asking both women their preference again, he discovered that the first had thought his day might have been so tiring that he would prefer dimly lit relaxation; the second had only been trying to tell him to be a little gentler.

No one can do everything right to please a partner. Even if every sexual move is fashioned to be absolutely gratifying, something in a lover's physical self will often be disturbing. We cannot be completely satisfied with one another. The secret lies in knowing what can be improved as opposed to what is unalterable.

Beyond what people can or can't tell one another about how they make love, myths about what great lovemaking should be may ruin postcoital satisfaction. Many people have fixed sexual standards that may not be violated. For some, foreplay, intercourse, and afterglow are the three unalterable sexual prerequisites. If any is lacking, they feel as though they have failed a significant test, or lost a contest. If an erection subsides, an orgasm fails to materialize, or an ejaculation occasionally lacks intensity, they worry with obsessional concern. Each act of intercourse becomes a ritual, like a tea ceremony. No room is allowed for the spillage, the broken china, and the surging appetites that may make passion so unexpectedly disastrous or marvelous.

Depending on character, too, all kinds of dramatic sexual expectations— intercourse as a pornographic charade, as a sentimental journey, or as a date with destiny—may be unmet. One can only suspect that union frequently destroys some aspect of another person's fantasy. Resentment collects during sex and emerges later.

The myth of the perfect relationship also reduces pleasure during and after sex. If people had to be absolutely attuned to one another's needs and wishes before sex, the act might never take place. But if two people are hostile to each other, they really shouldn't expect love to flow through the act. Some people, however, don't understand this basic rule of relationship. They make love because they feel they should, or because they think it will dissipate their anger. Feelings afterward may range from rage to disgust to humiliation.

Sometimes we can discover during sex that what has seemed a perfect relationship is actually fraught with unconscious difficulties. A woman will stop herself from pleasure during lovemaking for fear of being too intimately involved, dominated, rejected. A man will turn his love into aggressive sadism, or lose his erection, or fail to ejaculate because of some unconscious threat to his emotional security. These problems, of course, turn the postcoital bed into a white-sheeted wasteland of frustration or despair.

Feelings related to a partner's actual behavior after sex are a relatively new area for exploration and concern. This aspect of relationship may differ according to whether people are separating immediately after sex or spending the night, the weekend, or the rest of their lives. Whatever the case, the postcoital bed may reflect some sex-linked differences.

It takes fifteen or twenty minutes for women's vaginal mucosa to lose enough blood to return to normal color after climax. Therefore, I suspect, most women need fifteen or twenty minutes after the last orgasm to experience a sense of satisfied completion. Considering men who lose their erections quickly, I think many would be perfectly satisfied to rise from bed to get on with the day's activities immediately after depositing their contribution to immortality in the local receptacle. Many male mammals make vast courtship displays, engage in dominance battles with one another, and seduce with persistence worthy of any enamored swain, only to trot off with utter indifference after completing a sexual union. Maybe many men are just "that way" too—like horses.

What people who spend the rest of their lives together enjoy doing immediately after sex can be the cause of spoken or unspoken grievances, if they differ markedly. If they like remaining with one another, the first question is whether they want to continue coital emotions or change the subject. Do they want to elaborate the nuances of their love, or would getting up and making a big platter of bacon and eggs be more to the point? One woman patient was at her wit's end because just as she was usually ready to tell her husband how wonderful and loving their experience had been, he would suggest a ham sandwich and beer. Men do seem more eager than women to rush away from bed to other activities. Unaccustomed to feeling intimate, as one does during most passionate sexual engagements, or ashamed of the feeling, they try to avoid vulnerability afterward; they may go to sleep, get back to "work" with alacrity, raid the refrigerator, steep themselves in a book or TV program, or repair the sink.

Women tend to cry and complain more. The tears relate to the figurative abandonment after sex even though a partner may still be in bed; the complaints express the literal abandonment when a man returns to his preoccupation or his hobby, even though he remains "around the house."

Perhaps all these problems stand out in sharper relief when the lovemaking is short term and the couple must part soon after sexual intimacy. From "He just turns over and goes to sleep," the lament becomes, "He jumps up, wipes himself off with Kleenex, takes a shower, and runs."

Who rises from the coital bed first may be a matter of personality or politics. Many of my patients, both men and women, agree that it is most often the man. Even when the woman is confined by a tighter schedule, or the encounter is at "his place," or the exact time of separation is agreed in advance, the man will often more swiftly embrace the necessity for getting on with other realities. Politically, women often wait for men to take the lead in leave-taking as they used to wait for them to take the lead in initiating a relationship. Just as a woman may not have been willing to seem too forward, so she is often still unwilling to seem too self-sufficient. The "weaker sex" assumes the burden of taking rather than imposing rejection. The woman is the second person to stand up, if she gets up at all. This may be a matter of convenience if the tryst occurs at "her place," since she doesn't have to go anywhere and can afford to stay luxuriously in bed. The consensus in my acquaintance, however, is that men leave first under almost all circumstances.

Younger people tell me that more women are taking their leave without waiting for a signal, and I'm glad to hear it. One extremely independent friend with considerable sexual self-confidence reports that "it often works the other way around—when a man just 'wants' you to stay so badly, you feel burdened and constricted and want to get away." The tables are turning, and we can see new problems emerging as roles change and women start to do all sorts of things first. Perhaps the male need for affection was met in the past by knowing a woman didn't want him to leave. Perhaps female sexual lingering gave him, too, a sense of being busy, important, and in control. Perhaps when women do start to take the initiative, men will realize that they are not really like horses. They, too, crave affection. Maybe. Maybe not.

There are probably reasons for leaving first, or for going immediately to sleep, that are valid for either sex. If a partner is casual, one may wonder why on earth one has committed intimacy with this particular average specimen—this unexceptional male person in a polyester leisure suit, this female inanity who frizzed her hair because her hairdresser thought it would look smashing. It may seem urgent to leave quickly because mediocrity may be contagious, and lust has made us violate our better selves. Fleeing a one-time mate may signify only that he or she is not the stuff of dreams; the same haste in a long-standing relationship may indicate chronic unhappiness, emotional instability, or marriage to someone else.

The point at which we cannot tolerate another person's company for one more moment differs in all of us, and also differs depending on the person and the situation. When it's someone we don't care about, it comes sooner rather than later; when it's someone we love, we try to contain our impatience, but eventually the need for solitude, for privacy, for other company prevails. We must leave, or sleep, or read, or turn on music. We may go for a few minutes, an hour, a day, a year. The other person has been too noisy, too quiet, too passionate, too undemonstrative, too intellectual, too hysterical, too dry, too sentimental, too funny, too dour, and we can't give any more time. Away for a while, we will compose ourselves while our appetite is whetted again for the overwhelming flattery or the hard-to-get word of encouragement, the caressing tongue and hands. Long-term relationships are like that. One leaves in order to come back.

Whether the end of a particular experience of intercourse occurs between new lovers or familiar old consorts, certain psychological discords may always emerge. Distress may rise from the welter of one's internal struggles and include the old bugbears of guilt and shame for sexual pleasure itself. These interfere with an extraordinary number of coital acts and aftermaths. If one feels ashamed, sinful, exploited or otherwise soiled, demeaned, and dirty for one's sexual behavior, one can hardly descend from bed shining with innocent radiance. Guilt and shame induce depression.

Mood, too, plays a role in how people feel after sex. Two people can be in entirely disparate moods prior to intercourse and yet enjoy the coupling. Should they fail to perceive each other's dispositions, however, the aftermath can be a conflict. One partner may be gravely sober, contemplating a retreat to the grave, while a mate is amused at the absurdity of life. Or one may continue to be meshed in romantic illusion as the other presses to sustain reality. Other discords, less poetic, are more usual, leaving people stranded on their own existential islands, or at least alone on their own mental routes to the office, the supermarket, or the art gallery.

After sex, women more than men tend to be in touch with "postcoital *tristesse,*" feeling sad without precisely assigning a reason. In therapy, women most often trace this sadness to feelings of loss and separation. The closeness of intercourse is over. When a person feels sad about one parting, all other separations and losses seem to join the procession. People who have lost a significant relative, friend, teacher, or even another lover often mourn this loss after sexual intimacy. The reduction of boundaries when naked bodies merge may release conscious or unconscious memories. Some people are perfectly aware that they are remembering a grandmother's caress or a parent's tenderness; others are bewildered by the mystery and do not know what they are lamenting. The French expression for orgasm is "the little death." And after such a death we have the opportunity to mourn at our own gravesites. Resentment or depression can result when a lover ignores these feelings, runs away from them, negates them as "irrational," or tries to be cheery in the face of our penchant for grief.

Postcoital *tristesse* can be particularly strong when older people attempt to be more promiscuous than has always been comfortable for them; it may also be intense for young people when they embark on their sexual lives with a determination to achieve "experience" through variety. Sex does tend to activate emotional conduits in a great many people, notwithstanding all those who enjoy public practice without private feeling. People who do retain their sensibilities feel lost, abandoned, unhappy, lonely, and empty after such experiences. The problem is that they may think themselves defective for being melancholy.

Why do some people seem to feel nothing after sex? Why do others feel that their world is crushed like a tinsel ball when a lover leaves? Why do they fantasize death and destruction if he or she does not call the next day or keep a promise? Why do they sometimes kill themselves or others for loss of love, real or imagined? Postcoital feelings tell what a person's life—and what a relationship—is really about.

The Sofa, Rousseau, and Aphrodisia

MOHAIR VELVET UPHOLSTERY cloth cost $20 a yard when I bought it for my office sofa over twenty years ago. Recently I've been told it sells for $155 and is going up. Even at twenty it was high for me, but I bought it anyway. The reason I had to have a dark green mohair sofa was that the chair in which I sat on my grandfather's lap when I was a child was made of dark green mohair. If ever my patients were to grow to love one another, it would have to be upon the stiff yet soft fabric of my earliest affections.

Innumerable couples have sat on that sofa. Often they hold hands, as if they were dating, even as they ask me why the desire, the sex, and the lust has gone out of their marriage, why they are no longer "in love." They ask what switches they can pull to turn on the current again. Is there a "restart" button? Why have they become so ordinary to one another? Can they smoke, drink, or inhale anything, or can I write a prescription? Should they go to Tahiti, Tobago, Saint Thomas?

Lately, I have been ruminating a great deal about that sort of question because of the dust jacket of this book. While I was still in the process of setting down my thoughts, my publisher went ahead and prepared a jacket. It lies flat on a lamp table next to the mohair sofa in my office. The picture on it, a painting by Henri Rousseau called *The Snake Charmer*, hangs in the Louvre. Originally, I suggested using something by Gauguin, but my publisher was inspired to remember Rousseau. Gauguin went, as we all know, to Tahiti. Rousseau didn't go anywhere. Married to his beloved Clémence for several decades, he worked as a tax collector at the gates of Paris, copied wild animals from children's picture books, and haunted the local *jardin des plantes* for his exotic foliage.

I keep thinking that Henri Rousseau knew the answer to my couples' central question, and that it is related to the feeling I used to have when I sat on my grandfather Henry's lap on the mohair chair. Henry Fortgang was fat, warm, and sly. He liked to take my cheeks, one after the other, between his thumb and forefinger, and twist the flesh in what he said was the "Viennese" fashion. I would remain silent, bearing the pain as long as I could because it meant I could sit on his lap longer. Finally I would cry out. He would smile, release my cheek, and put me down. "Why don't you cry sooner?" he would always ask.

Rousseau stayed home. He had seven, possibly nine children. Two survived; the rest died in infancy. After his first wife died, he married again. His second wife died after four years. He had a few unsuccessful love affairs. He always asked the woman he courted to marry him. In a letter to the last, he wrote: "Whose fault is it if I am no use to you, from the point of view of cohabitation? Do you think I don't suffer? . . . Yes, you do make me suffer, for happily I still have my feelings. Let us unite and you will see if I am incapable of serving you." In the midst of the *fin de siècle* Parisian tumult—the Moulin Rouge, the can-

can, the Folies-Bergère, Sarah Bernhardt, and General Bou-
langer's midnight trysts—Henri Rousseau loved one woman at
a time and slept on the stairs outside his Léonie's door because
she would not let him in. Thinking upon Rousseau's pain and
his cocky, defensive posture against it, I conclude that he knew
the answer, and I suspect that the answer has something to do
with the feeling I had when I was hurt as a child. . . .

But let's clear the air and begin at the beginning. Let's be
logical. What is being "in love"? As a Supreme Court justice
once said of pornography, "I know it when I see it." But that's
not a very helpful definition. On one side of the experience,
most people want to be with their lover as much as possible. The
lover is a constant "presence," dreamed of, imagined, possessed,
sometimes imitated. They feel a tremendous energy, a release of
creativity, a high efficiency. Ordinary troubles are hardly disturbing. A constant eroticism pervades the love relationship and
almost all other activity, making pleasure continual and happiness a seemingly attainable goal.

On the underside of the passion is the hell of it. But without
uncertainty, fear of rejection, preoccupation with signs and por-
tents, and hope for reciprocity that will flood us with heaven,
falling in love would not have such deep, resonant power.

Why do we fall in love? No one precisely knows, except that
suffering often has something to do with it.

The distress may result from one of life's predictable transitions, most often that of leaving one's family for the first time.
As normal as the separation may be, it can be painful, and the
pain can be the catalyst for falling in love. On the other side of
the door, parents experiencing the difficulties of parting with
their children may find new love for one another, or go their own
ways to new lovers. Whether one leaves or is left, fresh love may
come along.

A grimmer pain is caused by grief and mourning. Some studies of marital statistics have shown new loves to rise, as it were, from recent graves. Often within a year, people marry to refill the emptiness created in their lives by the death of a husband or wife, a parent, or even a sibling. We repair our wounds, replace our losses.

Deprivation, if not too intense, may also stimulate love. If we are in situations that keep us from friendly human contact—long work on a solitary project, a prolonged time alone in meditation, an intense involvement in the heavy negotiation of the world's business—emergence from the deprived state may ready us for love.

The dream of perfect union may arise, too, from conscious and unconscious memories of our infancy and early childhood. The wish for dependence, fusion, and mastery-under-guidance may lead to an imaginary ideal state where we totally rely on one another for all warm feelings. We dream of cooperating in the tasks of life, our mutual support eliminating stress. We want to protect one another against the intrusion of the world's problems. Together, we try to keep out the philistine ugliness, the disease of pragmatism, the insatiable demands of other people's rituals. We are a fortress against the enemy. We join one another, and in so doing, we complete ourselves.

Falling in love, of course, may include sexual longings and sexual relations, but not always specifically. It is as though all acts performed together are the equivalent of intercourse. A visit to an art gallery, a meal together, or a browse about a bookstore might feel as much like making love as actual physical union. All of life is eroticized, not merely the sexual moment. During the acute phase of joy, however, sex is usually experienced as wonderful, whether the mechanics are precisely right or not and often even if a couple is actually unsuited.

Why, then, do people fall "out of love"? With that fine

start, why does it so often go stale and dry?

Much about the state of being "in love" does imitate illusory madness. The person we adore cannot possibly be so adorable; being with him or her perpetually could not be an eternal idyll; the presence or imagined presence of a beloved does not eliminate despair or incompetence. Certainly, if a lover is sexually limited, we cannot continue to delude ourselves about his or her abilities forever.

At a simplistic level, perhaps being in love lasts as long as one can maintain the illusion. As soon as the great placebo wears off, pain must be faced again. Just as we all have varying capacities for obsession—the loved one occupying anywhere from 20 to 99.9 percent of our waking thought—so we have a varying capacity for fantasy and illusion. Some people sustain imaginary joy for a lifetime; others can make it last only an hour. People at the ends of the spectrum live what seem to be difficult lives. Changing love objects once every few months, or even once a year, would seem as difficult and unsettling as having to continually sell one's house and move to a different part of town. Some people, however, can only survive by sequential diversity, just as others can only love once. Among the saddest stories I ever heard was that of a man who loved only once, and then for but three days.

It may be that the euphoria is meant to sustain one until sex and procreation get under way. We—particularly women—may be programmed to fall in love so that we will assume the immense undertaking of giving birth without caring about its pain or the travails of parenthood. I have heard it said that we may be similarly programmed for death, our bodies infused at the last with naturally euphoriant chemicals to ease our passage through the gates of heaven.

Some authorities feel that being "in love" lasts until "brood behavior" is established, most often in two years time. After that, the parents may go on to a more realistic affection or to a separation. These days, the high divorce rate among parents with young children testifies to early disillusion. It seems to validate our ancestors' insistence on economic and other sensible bonds for matrimony. Given free choice and free rein, we appear to be more careless of our attachments than we would like to believe ourselves to be.

Ideally, as we all know because the tale has been told by millions of folk tongues for centuries, we fall in love and then grow to know and care for each other in time. The consummation of marriage reassures us of our bonds, and we need no longer live in fear of loss. Falling in love has precipitated a larger relationship where affection may increase between people and nourish the lives that it produces.

I do not think I have to retell the fairy tale any further, though it always makes people feel good to hear about "happily ever after." Sometimes people really do create the marriage of their dreams as they work their way beyond the obsession, the illusion. More often, people fall out of love. It is usually a slow process of which the participants are unaware until one day the inescapable emotional fact appears in their consciousness, perhaps abruptly at breakfast. No more dreams. No more luminosity. The shores of marble and the rivers of chalcedony are gravel and sludge. "Please pass the salt." "Do you think you could chew your toast more quietly, love?" The couple leave the breakfast table and come to sit on my sofa. They don't really want each other anymore, but they've signed a contract. Maybe if the sex were better, life together would be more attractive.

One of the first things I often do is to help them define what they have lost, at least sexually. Oddly enough, they usually accept that the grander illusions cannot return; everyone seems to know that. They dismiss their dreams as "puppy love." We agree that illusions must be channeled elsewhere, perhaps ultimately to our expectations of an afterlife. We laugh maturely about that.

Sexually, I explain, they seem fragmented; their desire and their excitement appear to be cut off from each other. Desire, the wish to have sex, and excitement, the physical response to that wish, have been separated. We may not be able to put them together again with any great heat of reaction, any cataclysmic hiss as the chemicals unite, but we may be able to accomplish a pleasant mix, a warm solution.

Desire may be understood as an intellectual state. One can say, "I want to have sex," meaning, "I like the idea of erotic relations." At the time of this statement, one need not be experiencing excitement. Indeed, one could be eating cucumber slices during the television commercial and merely reflecting a philosophical generality. Or one could also say to a friend, who might be munching on oranges, "I want to have sex with Harry," thus making the object more specific. Neither statement implies any genital oscillations, any lubricating or erectile activity. Yet both express what we (scientifically, anyway) call "desire."

Excitement, on the other hand, refers to any pleasurable physical commotion caused by the thought of having sex. It also refers to the body changes that occur during sexual activity.

If a boy has a sexual fantasy and finds himself erect, he is in a state of excitement. If a girl is doing her homework and experiences a genital signal that makes her want to masturbate for tension relief, she has become excited. If a couple are making love, with tenderness, joy, lust, and considerable athletic vigor, they are excited. When the sex organs, the heart, the lungs, and the sweat glands are all working away together, more actively than usual, a state of excitation prevails.

Most people make the error, however, of thinking that desire and excitement follow each other sequentially, like the numbers *one* and *two* or the letters *A* and *B.* While this may happen, the more usual state of affairs is for both to occur together, almost simultaneously. The thought of having sex with Harry, the desire to do so, elicits an excitement response in Jane. Or an excitement response occurs in Harry while he is riding on a bumpy bus, and elicits the desire to have sex with Jane. Either way, the two are merely ingredients of the sexual reaction.

Just as desire may be experienced without excitement, so excitement can occur without desire. A woman may experience excitement during sexual relations without any desire to have intercourse. Many women have the ability to be passively aroused without particularly willing any union, although consent is necessary. Over the centuries, this particular gift has caused a great deal of confusion and trouble. A woman's consent may be mistaken for desire and her aroused response construed as excited enjoyment. In my practice I've found that many women are capable of having excited, orgasmic sex without desire or emotional pleasure. Many can also be brought to excitement and orgasm when all they start with is desire. Men without desire may be led by their erections to intercourse. Men without excitement cannot perform.

Rarely have I encountered a patient who has lost all desire; most people want to have sex, at least in the philosophic sense. A failure of the capacity for excitement is not common among my patients either. I think we would find, on testing, that their genitals react frequently even during sleep to messages from the brain, cyclically erecting or lubricating. What couples seem to lose in the long struggle, or the long tedium, of living together is the simultaneous occurrence of desire and excitement. When the wish for sex and sexual arousal are strong and closely related, people enter a state of aphrodisia. They long for consummation. They appreciate even the lightest touch. They desire and are excited at the same time. They may want to be together after sex, too, which is perhaps the most distinctive feature of the aphrodisia of being in love, as compared to sexual infatuation.

What fractures aphrodisia? What breaks the union between desire and excitement, and what can we do about it?

The most common source of aphrodisia, whether that of sexual infatuation or being in love, is novelty. For a great many human beings, novelty is as aphrodisiac as it was to those rodents who, in lab tests, experienced a significant increase in testosterone level and a great eagerness for sexual relations when new females were placed in their cages, even though the old ones were still there. (I find it most appropriate that men who engage in a sexual pattern of several intense encounters and then lose interest are frequently known as "rats.")

In women, the factor that seems to contribute to aphrodisia most is fear—precisely the right amount to evoke a "thrill." Rather like the joy of riding a roller coaster, skiing down a mountain, or hang-gliding, the various emotional thrills related to sex offer a powerful motive for pleasure to erotic novitiates as well as a continuing stimulus to the confirmed erotic sportsperson. For both men and women, fear and novelty, or fear plus novelty, produce precisely the right challenge to create a temporary aphrodisia.

These two elements must inevitably abate. We experience less excitement with a mate to whom we are accustomed. That is the way of the world. Couples sometimes need to be told that they will never be excitingly new to each other again. If sex is distinctly unpleasant, however, something else is probably wrong. Even diminished pleasures ought to be pleasant enough to seek and enjoy.

Of course there is such a thing as too much fear. Sometimes people are so afraid of sex, or intimacy, or any of the basic functions that they try to keep a relationship blooming on the thin stalk of cerebration. Revulsion occurs at the prospect of enjoying earthy pleasure. The flower dies. Aphrodisia ceases in the face of simple naked reality.

Most commonly, however, anger is the great cause of falling out of love. Some people become only accurately angry; others, which is to say most of us, become angry at the perception of any threat, real or not. To the psychiatrist, the word *anger* implies not only any overt demonstration of rage, but any nuance of the feeling, from hidden and unspoken resentment to violent explosion. Indeed, more damage is generally done to aphrodisia by our quiet retaliations than by our upheavals of discontent.

We destroy our happiness with the same tools that we use to destroy ourselves and one another. Personality is a major factor in the fate of sexual attraction over time. How we handle anger, how suspicious-trusting, generous-greedy, dominant-submissive, lively-indolent we are, and how our mates feel about these qualities may lead to the longevity or the demise of sexual feeling.

When a couple marry, one of their first problems is territoriality. Resolving needs for privacy, ownership, and space create considerable dissension. The birth of children deals a further blow to sexuality. Jealousies are aroused: Baby gets attention, a spouse loses it. Anger is unexpected, felt to be unjustified, but nevertheless persists. The man or the woman may then deem it time to make the big career push. Again, neglect and rage, suppressed by reasonable people, afflict the marriage bed. The person attempting to get ahead suffers anxiety and insecurity. The partner feels abandoned. So it goes through all the trials: children's illnesses, parents' deaths, and the next stress and the next, good or bad, profitable or not, driving people apart.

Rather than being surprised at the reduction in sex drive, I am surprised that any remains at all among people bound to one another for better or for worse. So much in life is worse. And it is so much easier, at least for mobile urban people, to remove their libido from the scene of household frustration or tragedy and place it with transitory lovers who may be discarded at the first hint of trouble.

On a social level, women's continuing economic inequality may hamper aphrodisia. Faced with the necessity of proving themselves in a world where men have made it difficult to do so, many women experience a slow or sudden onset of sexual anomie. The anxiety of the quest and new convictions about men as enemies may take a high toll of sexual energy. The wife who suddenly realizes that identification with her husband has not solved her own identity problem, who starts to wonder where her collegiate persona has gone, or who suddenly must work at a debasing job for financial reasons makes an excellent candidate for hostility, depression, and loss of libido.

Whatever the source, anger—expressed or unexpressed— rarely promotes love and sexual fervor. Some modern psychological theorists seem to encourage us to exist in a constant temper tantrum. I would venture that people who flail, cry, yell, beat walls, and threaten to do one another in generally do not experience a freer sexuality than those who case themselves in emotional steel, boil inside, and feel too hot to touch. Whether a couple's anger is spoken or withheld, broadcast or censored, made visible or hidden, I take it as my crucial concern—and theirs—to resolve the issue.

Many people have had the experience of feeling sexually liberated after expressing bottled-up rage. They feel free for the first time in a long time, or even ever. When I began working with such people, particularly women, I mistakenly credited the anger with the cure. Actually, something in our therapeutic transaction probably made the person feel sufficiently self-confident to take a stand. The new self-esteem, rather than the destructive explosion, freed sexual response. During emotional stress, when people feel aggressive or fearful, sexual relations rarely head the priority list.

Only in serious sexual deviation does a man use his penis as a weapon of attack. Although both sexes can and do use lust as an expression of malice or contempt, I do not usually encourage this aspect of sexual relationship. I prefer to labor in behalf of peace—and freedom from anger, anguish, and anxiety—as the source and the goal of sexual feelings in marriage.

Indeed, one of the most misleading contemporary beliefs I've encountered is that anger resembles steam in a pressure cooker, needing to be let out, or liquid in a container that can be emptied. May I suggest that rage, like the red light on the dashboard, signals trouble that needs attending to. Too much anger in a marriage points to something wrong either with the relationship or with one or both of the partners.

Perhaps the most difficult anger to deal with starts outside the marriage. Like children becoming angry at their parents when frustrated by a teacher, mates often whip their spouses with anger generated at another source. This kind of anger devastates sex most effectively, since it cannot be resolved until the outside problem abates.

The people who hold hands on my couch seldom feel their anger overtly, if at all. They tend to believe that tolerance is an aspect of civilized manners and restraint an indicator of charac-ter. Unfortunately, they often stretch the concept of good man-ners to the point of noncommunication. For good sex as for good living, I believe that repressing a problem is not much use. To live well with one another as adults, we must learn to verbalize our difficulties, our hurts, and our rages in such a way that a partner may recognize their existence and understand their cause. When conflict is resolved, sex may return and become trusting and loving again.

Beyond these angers are the discords that accompany the

emergence of individual character as a marriage proceeds. While in love, we give ourselves entirely to our partners. Soon, however, sometimes very soon, we become "selfish." We may return to our solitary hobbies, read the newspapers, follow sports, prefer silence to conversation, or elect to discuss politics with a friend rather than declare our nightly amour. We begin to individuate, in the same way that children go through phase after phase of differentiating themselves from their parents and siblings. We, too, separate again, this time from our mates. We express our tastes, confess our distastes. Occasionally we find, even after believing otherwise for years, that we are living with or married to someone who might have been born on another planet, for all the community of interest that truly exists. Sometimes opposite temperaments and talents spark sexuality. More often, they destroy it. Recreation may become impossible as the nondancers battle the music while their partners wither in frustration, or as movie lovers fall asleep too often at the opera, or as beach-persons suffer claustrophobia at mountain retreats. He reads mystery stories; she likes biography. She despises cooking; he attends classes in Chinese cuisine. In my work with one couple, all I could find of mutual interest was the ability to ride a bicycle. It wasn't quite enough to save their sex life.

At a specifically erotic level, too, differences emerge that may not have been at all obvious at the start. One of the most prevalent is the approach to sex and pornography. In a relationship, often many men are unable to be stimulated except by the pornographic scenarios to which they have become conditioned. Many women remain minimally exposed to and maximally repelled by these stimulants. Under these conditions, love frequently continues but sex fails, with currents of rage seething beneath the marital coverlet. She wonders why he can't respond to warmth, love, and music; he wonders why she won't become sexually flamboyant so they can have "real sex." While pornography has always existed, it used to be secret, expensive, and not present enough in men's lives to be necessary. Now, many men—and women—cannot do without it. Cheap and plentiful, like junk food, it is part of our culture and makes up an extraordinary percentage of the national diet.

More functionally, specific sexual difficulties emerge. Suddenly it is clear that a man is so sexually sensitive that intercourse is too brief to give the woman orgasmic satisfaction. Or he needs vigorous stimulation and she thinks sex is best while lying still. Or she has been "faking" orgasms to prove her love and protect his "ego," but now she has begun to feel deprived.

People's psyches may prevent their admitting, much less solving, these problems. An interesting aspect of liberation involved a case where a woman could not have orgasms with her boss, who was also—incidentally—her husband. She was multiorgasmic, however, with men in the organization who ranked below her. She could not tell "Daddy" what she wanted or what to do, but functioned very well with subordinates. This is quite reminiscent of men who are impotent with all but witless women.

The point is that after being "in love" wears off, reality often discloses both personal and sexual defects and characteristics. To improve the relationship, to establish a true community of interest or real sexual rapport, may take quite a long time and a great deal of honest hard labor.

I do not believe that the world is suffering a new sexual cancer. Marital sex was never perpetually aphrodisiac. One is hard pressed to recall any historical era of perfect marriage. Sex has been traditionally lusty among people seeking novelty or adventure, and frequently workaday, placid, and even dull between accustomed mates. The difference is that with our new psychological tools and insights, we have discovered ways to decrease anger and therefore to increase love between old lovers. We "improve communication." We can help people say simply to one another what they feel, without undue fear of retaliation. We can help them to speak of the sensitive privacies of their sexual life, tell the hidden hurts and happinesses. When we understand one another, we can often forgive, begin again, change.

Of Rousseau, Paul Eluard wrote, "We are fortunate that, in his naïveté, Henri Rousseau was convinced that he must show us what he saw. What he saw was love, and he will always make us look at the world through enchanted eyes." Another critic wrote that "what Rousseau restores to us is nothing less than an eternal human longing for a lost Eden."

I think that what I have been trying to say is that pain is a universal condition over which we have some small controls. We can cry out now and then, and the devil, like my old grandfather, may stop pinching our cheeks. We can lessen the pain more permanently by falling in love with life.

Acknowledgments

THE WRITER, like the psychiatrist, traditionally works alone. Yet craft and inspiration must be supported. I am indebted to family, teachers, colleagues, friends, and patients. I have acknowledged my family in the lines of this book. For their rich and various contributions to my professional experience, and though some of them are no longer here to accept my gratitude, I originally thanked:

Dr. Hugh R.K. Barber, Dr. John Astrachan, Dr. Sidney Kreps, Dr. Harry Fein, Dr. Thomas Argyros, Dr. Colter Rule, Dr. Seymour Grossman, Dr. Lawrence Downs, Dr. Mary DiGangi, Dr. William Frosch, Dr. Damir Velcek, Dr. Howard Bogard, Dr. Don Sloan, Dr. Lisa Tallal, Dr. Michael Bruno, Dr. Harvey Klein, Dr. David Jacobs, Dr. Marilyn Karmason, Dr. Louis Wolfe, Dr. Maj-Britt Rosenbaum, Dr. Eric Carlson, Dr. Jacques Quen, Dr. Lenard Jacobson, Dr. Richard Glass, Dr. Wayne Myers, Dr. Robert Kaye, Dr. Ruth Bruun, Dr. Alvin Donnenfeld, Dr. Lawrence Hatterer, Dr. John Williams, Dr. Patrizia Levi, Dr. Garwood Leckband, Dr. Murray Silver, Dr.

James Kocsis, Dr. Howard Wiener, Dr. Loren Skeist, Dr. Kurt Adler, Dr. Alfred Ainbinder, Dr. Stanley Birnbaum, Dr. Norman Deane, Dr. Robert Michels, Dr. Allen Collins, Dr. David James, Dr. Ruth Cohen, Dr. Maurice Carter, Dr. Nicholas Pace, Dr. Wayne Decker, Dr. Helen Klein, Dr. Herbert Kupperman, Dr. Morrison Levbarg, Dr. Hugh Melnick, Dr. Daniel Neyman, Dr. Anthony Orlando, Dr. Borisse Paulin, Dr. George Weingarten, Dr. Fred Snyder, Dr. Stuart Orsher, Dr. George McLemore, Dr. Francis Kane, Dr. Daniel Hartman, Dr. Doris Nagel, and Dr. Robert Halsband.

Candida Donadio and her associate Melanie Jackson were the first to represent me as literary agents with special patience for the vagaries of my dual career. It is a tribute to my initial publisher, Thomas Congdon, and his versatile editor, Gretchen Salisbury, that their attentions made us better friends. Now I thank especially Jason Aronson, Diane Turek, Ruth E. Brody and Michael Moskowitz for their patience with my revisions as this book once again goes to press to satisfy my gentle readers, old and new.

—A.O.

Index

249

About the Author

Avodah K. Offit, M.D., has written two other books, both of which have been acclaimed widely as eloquent and, indeed, brilliant. Her most recent is *Virtual Love,* an E-mail novel about two psychiatrists, published by Simon & Schuster in 1994. Kurt Vonnegut wrote, "Avodah Offit joins the small company of able physicians who are born storytellers as well, in her case spinning erotic tales in the voice of what she is in real life, a wise and profoundly experienced sex therapist."

Dr. Offit's first book, *The Sexual Self,* was described by the *Times* as "wonderful, strewn with wit and insight and written with compassion and sensibility." This collection of essays has been translated into French, German, and Spanish editions. She has also contributed chapters to various textbooks and articles to many magazines.

The author is a graduate of Hunter College and the University of Chicago. She majored in English and was elected to Phi Beta Kappa. She graduated from the New York University School of Medicine and is in the private practice of psychiatry and sex therapy. A consultant at Lenox Hill Hospital, she holds her clinical academic professorship at Cornell University Medical College in affiliation with the New York Hospital.

Her online address is: Virtualove@aol.com.